FOR A REASON

VALERIE,

RESILIENCE BEGINS WITH A REASON.
THANK YOU FOR YOUR FRIENDSHIP &
SUPPORT.

LOVE ALWAYS,

Hope
Survivorship
Community
Determination
Resilience

BY DANNY HEINSOHN

Cover Design & Layout: Access Pass & Design, Bill Nutt
Cover Photo Credit: Margie Webb

ISBN: 978-0-9900168-0-9

Primary editing contribution by Mike Urban
Content feedback contributions by Sherre Frost, Tiffany Thiele, Dan
Carlstrom, and Gene Kim
Page design layout by Ponderosa Pine Design, Vicky Vaughn Shea

Printed in China by Regent Publishing Services Ltd.

*Disclaimer: Information in this book is based on hands-on experience. The
author is not a trained professional in any health, environmental, or other
field; he will not be responsible for the consequences of the application of any
information or ideas presented herein.*

Dedication

To the loving memory of my dad, Ted Heinsohn.

To my mom who always makes things better, Kimberly Heinsohn.

And to all friends and family who have inspired and supported
me over the years.

SPECIAL THANKS TO . . .

Book cover design by Bill Nutt.

Primary editing contributions by Mike Urban.
Assisted editing contributions by Sherre Frost, Tiffany Thiele,
Dan Carlstrom & Gene Kim.

Page layout design contribution by Vicky Vaughn Shea.

CONTENTS

PART TWO – THE YEARS

PREFACE

Life is truly what you make of it. Who would have thought that after being diagnosed with brain cancer at the age of 23, surviving three craniotomies, and enduring a year of chemotherapy, that I would end up working with the biggest names in sports and entertainment? Then ten years later, who would've thought that I'd start my own foundation and finish an Ironman triathlon in less than 12 hours to celebrate the decade milestone of being cancer free? I believe that prosperity will always follow passion, and when you have passion nothing can stand in your way.

Surviving brain cancer and enduring the trials after treatment illuminated the most important things in life during my mid-twenties. While many young adults graduate college, begin their careers, join the military, or travel, I was in for the fight of my life.

Recovering from three brain surgeries, losing my memory, losing my ability to speak, read and write, dealing with seizures, enduring twelve months of chemotherapy, overcoming depression, learning the art of letting go, and believing in myself again were all milestones I met as a young adult. But none of those milestones came easy and nothing came without sacrifice and perseverance; especially for my mom and dad. I am an only child.

Life during cancer treatment wasn't easy. In fact things could've very well taken a turn for the worse many times. Every day of surgery or chemotherapy had a mortality risk factor. When treatment was over there were no guarantees my cancer was gone for good. But through the toughest of times, I immediately realized that the beauty of life is through the love, compassion, and support of friends, family, and the community. They made me feel like the luckiest person in the world. They were my heroes and inspired me to become the person I am today.

When everything is on the line luck may be the only thing going for you. Whether it's through someone you know, something you observe, something you realize, or something that happens, luck can change the course of a less favorable outcome. Life or death, win or lose, success or failure, luck plays a role in the outcome. Everyone needs luck to catch a break. Luck is what happens when we try harder, give more, or surround ourselves with the right people.

I am a brain cancer survivor and I am lucky to be alive. The circumstances and the people who cared for and treated me as I endured treatment created all the luck I needed to live a productive life. In what could have been a prognosis of less than five years to live, has so far turned out to be over a decade.

Although I don't categorize myself to any particular religious faith, I do believe in love, hope, community, determination, and resilience. Those are the beliefs I feel everyone can relate to. Those beliefs have given me a reason to live my life with courage and conviction. Through the compassion, love and support of others, I found a reason to keep pressing forward and setting an example of what it means to be a brain cancer survivor.

Ever since I was diagnosed with brain cancer at the age of 23, my life has been all about determination and perseverance. I've never given up on an opportunity I believed in and always believed I could do better or do more. This is one of the blessings that came through living life during and after cancer. You name it, marathons, century bike rides, triathlons, sports marketing, becoming an author and public speaker; the people who know me best know that I will find a way.

I also learned that no one succeeds alone. People need people to network, help overcome hardships, and advance through life. After finishing a year of chemotherapy my motives for making money weren't as relevant than when I was going through college. Money was important to make a living but my drive was to find a way to help people and make a difference. I realized the significance of this when support came pouring in before the doctors and nurses opened my skull to remove a racquetball size tumor.

My friends and family were my anchor and my reason to live. I couldn't let them down.

There is something to be said about the determination and grit that the hardships of a cancer diagnosis brings. In my professional life I have found a way to work with the biggest names in sports and entertainment. I've been lucky, but I've also gotten to be really good at what I do. In fact I have created some amazing opportunities through a career that has enabled me to work with the New York Yankees, Baltimore Ravens, The Rolling Stones, Jason Mraz, Ben Harper, The Black Keys, Nevada Wolf Pack, and the Chicago Blackhawks.

In my personal life I found healing and a passion through endurance sports. I am an Ironman Triathlete, finisher of over 50 triathlons, centuries, and marathons, and am a former cycling coach.

My friends and family sometimes ask when I'm going to take a break and settle down. Truth is I've tried, and I do. But my idea of taking a break is spending a week in Alaska, the Galapagos Islands, or Costa Rica while packing in whitewater rafting, waterfall repelling, sockeye fly fishing, swimming with marine life, and hiking volcanoes. By the time I return home and recover, I'm recharged, ready to train for my next race or ready to hop on a plane and stir up business opportunities with corporate brands and sports properties.

I've spent nearly 14 years writing this book. It began with an essay I wrote not long after I was diagnosed in 1999, followed by several journal entries throughout the years. But there would be years without any writing at all because living my life and building a career became more important than constantly reflecting on the past. But eventually I made the commitment to finish the book after my tenth year of remission, after I finished Ironman Canada and founded my own charity organization.

This book is about my life before, during, and after cancer. Living through cancer made me who I am today, and every day I'm motivated by what it has taught me. Pursue your dreams, help others, and never give up.

INTRODUCTION

The draft for the Vietnam War was instituted during the Nixon administration in 1969. My dad was born in 1948 and was of prime age at the time. His draft number ranked low, which meant it was only a matter of time before he would be called to action.

Around that same time, his father died of a stroke at the age of 49. My grandfather was a medic during World War II who smoked like chimney and was a chronic caffeine drinker. At this time of uncertainty my dad quickly assessed his options and decided to join the army himself to avoid the draft, and he was soon shipped to Korea, where he met my mom in 1974.

I was born on February 5, 1976, in Fort Ord, California. That same year Steve Jobs and Steve Wozniak started Apple, Jimmy Carter was elected president, the Summer Olympics were held in Montreal, Bob Marley was shot in Kingston, Jamaica, and a band called U2 was formed in Dublin. My grandmother would pass away from colon cancer at the age of 52, a couple years after I was born.

I grew up in Reno, Nevada. In the 1980s I remember the news of the Mount St. Helens eruption. My parents bought an Atari computer for Christmas in 1981. The movie *E.T.* was released in 1982, along with Michael Jackson's *Thriller*. Bruce Springsteen's album *Born in the USA* debuted in 1984, and the Summer Olympics were held in Los Angeles. In 1986 NASA's space shuttle *Challenger* disintegrated on live TV, and the Boston Red Sox choked in the World Series. *The Goonies, Raiders of the Lost Ark*, and *Ghostbusters* were among my favorite movies, while *MacGyver, The A-Team*, and *Night Court* ranked high on my primetime TV shows list.

As a teenager, I found social identity through playing sports, collecting baseball cards, and listening to rap, R&B, and heavy metal music. I graduated high school in 1994, travelled to Mazatlan, Mexico, for my senior class trip, and watched OJ Simpson get arrested on live TV while drinking Pacifico beer.

By the time I got to college, my dreams of becoming a professional baseball player had dissolved. I forged a new path by pledging the Pi Kappa Alpha fraternity, where I could still stay competitive in intramural sports, build a professional network for my future, and enjoy the social benefits of Greek life. A year later my taste in music evolved, and I felt liberated with the discovery of punk rock and driving to California to watch live concerts with my friends during the summer and winter breaks.

A lot of great things were in alignment upon entering my final year of college. I was elected college of engineering senator the spring before and worked to implement a mentor program for incoming freshman. I was maintaining an above-average GPA, had a great resume, left school early to ski on Friday afternoons, and occasionally played open mic guitar nights with my buddies.

After changing majors three times, I graduated with a Bachelor of Science degree in Electrical Engineering in May 1999. The plan after college graduation was to backpack around Europe for two and a half months with two of my best friends, move to Colorado or Arizona to begin my professional career, and live the life of an eligible bachelor.

The day after I graduated, brain cancer came into my life like a storm front. Upon arrival it consumed my family and tested us in ways we could never imagine. Life had lessons to teach.

PART ONE

The Months

CHAPTER 1

A CHILLING BREEZE

SATURDAY – MAY 8, 1999

One day until my last final and eight days from completing my college undergraduate curriculum. I was twenty-three and thankful to be on the brink of college graduation. The culmination of five college years seemed to fly by like a flock of migrating geese to a more prosperous wetland. I most certainly yearned for a change of culture and opportunities to explore new ones. The plan after graduation was a two-month European backpack excursion with two of my best friends, whom I have known since childhood. Elation began to take hold, and commencement was the final step before the next phase of my life.

SUNDAY - MAY 9

At approximately 10 a.m. I awakened to a beautiful morning. Anticipation enthralled me, similar to feelings I experienced in elementary school the day before summer vacation. After rolling out of bed to stir around my apartment, a sharp headache lingered behind my left eyeball. I thought, "Maybe I'm not hydrated efficiently." Not taking much concern at all, I got out of bed, skipped taking a shower, ate breakfast, drank two glasses of water, packed my books, walked down the stairs of my apartment, stepped into my 4x4 extended cab pickup truck, and started the engine. I drove to a computer lab, where I would rendezvous with a study group and begin reviewing for the last final of our undergraduate college careers. Bittersweet thoughts came to mind; I wasn't done yet, but after one last day of studying and one more long final, I would be.

"No more classes, no more books, no more teacher's dirty looks," a verse well remembered from Bugs Bunny in *Looney Toons* cartoons. In less than twenty-four hours, I would be singing my own version. No more labs, no more verbal presentations, no more study groups, no more student senate meetings, no more cramming for finals, no more homework, no more quizzes, no more luncheons.

I crammed and reviewed for six hours throughout the course of the day and into the evening. Meanwhile something peculiar was upsetting my conventional way of thinking. As I walked to and from my truck, up and down the hallways to lab, and back and forth to the restroom, a persistent pressure lingered behind my left eyeball. After a rigorous day of reviewing my notes, I thought, "Everything will be fine in the morning," and I fell into a comfortable slumber.

MONDAY – MAY 10

I awakened with another bothersome headache, ate a bagel, drank a tall glass of water, and drove to a different computer lab where the final was to take place. I struggled through the irritation to complete my last final in a course called Digital Control Systems. It was difficult to decide if I wanted to blame the overwhelming difficulty of the exam or the irritation in my head. I finished in an agonizing fashion, both mentally and neurologically.

Upon exiting the computer lab, many of my peers were congregated in the hall. Our curriculum was one of the most challenging at the university, and we always waited for each other outside the exam room to discuss or ridicule the tough problems. This exam was no different; but instead of discussing the difficult problems, we expressed sighs of relief that it was our last final. Still, my head felt like twisted metal as I painfully tried to unveil my thoughts. It hurt to think . . . it hurt to shake my head . . . all day long.

TUESDAY – MAY 11

Another awful headache welcomed me as I rose from my bed in the morning. I decided to call a doctor and set an appointment as soon as possible;

the next available time slot was two days later. On that very evening I began to notice something was very wrong as I ran the base paths during a softball game. With each stride it felt as if a river rock rattled in my head, particularly behind my left eyeball. The discomfort was excruciating.

A week from this day, the itinerary for the next two months of my life would be a tour around Europe. The adventure was to begin in Bilbao, Spain, then extend throughout much of the continent. I certainly didn't want to have a rock in my head while overseas. Although I never experienced anything like it, I was optimistic that the disturbance was something temporary.

WEDNESDAY – MAY 12

I opened my eyes, feeling normal, but the same unwanted nuisance remained as I raised my torso. The instability in my head was like two positively charged magnets repelling each other. To be redundant, I scheduled another appointment for the upcoming Friday, in search of a second opinion.

THURSDAY – MAY 13

At my first appointment, a doctor from a local medical clinic told me that the headaches were likely caused by the stress of finals, anxiety to graduate, and the impending trip to Europe. Knowing myself and my health, I didn't buy it, and my concern became suspicion. Graduating and travelling to Europe were exciting things to look forward to but nothing to get a pounding headache over. Don't get me wrong, I had episodes of sensory overload throughout college, but those came with the territory. I was experiencing an intense throbbing. Despite my circumstance, I remained confident that it would pass within the next few days. I received two prescriptions to reduce my symptoms. "If symptoms continue, call us back." You know the routine. Hopefully the doc was right.

Upon leaving the parking lot, I backed into a FedEx delivery truck and busted my driver-side taillight. No harm was done to the FedEx truck, but I wondered, "How could my depth perception be so shallow?"

FRIDAY, SATURDAY – MAY 14, 15

Friday was the same story as Thursday. Saturday the headaches subsided slightly, perhaps from the antibiotics.

SUNDAY, MAY 16 – COMMENCEMENT

After five fast and crazy years as a student at the University of Nevada, I received my validation of hard work and accomplishment. It was a beautiful day but boring to sit nearly four hours while hundreds graduated. At least my fellow graduating classmates and I were able to pass the time with jokes as we sat through the tediousness. Meanwhile, my attention was primarily focused on *Europe Through the Back Door* by Rick Steves. I bought it after my roommate, Brian Moynihan, suggested it weeks earlier.

I did it, Bachelor of Science in Electrical Engineering, and I was more relieved than ever. Besides my peers, my primary spectators were family members: Aunt Melva, Aunt Sherre, Aunt Betty, Uncle Marvin, Uncle Sid, Cousin Don, Cousin Windy, and my loving father and mother, Ted and Kim. They beamed with pride. Within forty-eight hours, I would be on my way to Europe for a two-month vacation.

My head pounded all day with each agonizing step, but I managed to mask the discomfort with forced smiles and a calm demeanor. *What was going on?* That night we all gathered for a family dinner at a casino buffet to cap my celebration of perseverance. Everybody was jubilant except for the rock in my head.

CONGRATULATIONS

This scroll is in commemoration of the commencement activities conducted this day in Reno, Nevada. Your participation in this ceremony signifies the formal ending of one very important part of your life and the beginning of another. You are to be commended and congratulated for this accomplishment. May all your hopes and high aspirations for the future be as richly rewarding as this achievement.

11

College Spring Break - March 15-20, 1999

Two months prior to graduation, I enjoyed my last and most pleasurable college spring break in Oahu, Hawaii. The air was fresh, the culture laid back, and I was happy, livin' life, and lovin' every moment. For a week, I was in paradise with three of my friends from student senate. It was Dave White and Jesse Viner, who were College of Arts and Science senators, and Mike Bowers, who represented the College of Journalism. Mike was also speaker of the senate, while I was one of two College of Engineering senators. The four of us were in our own element, happy to break away from the usual college grind.

None of us had ever been to Hawaii, but we had a pretty good idea of what we wanted to do when we got there: party, hook up with coeds, and relax. Items on the to-do list included marlin fishing, snorkeling in Hanauma Bay, explore the island by way of moped, a booze cruise, and of course, surfing, all of which were accomplished. The everyday, arduous tasks of demanding college life became obsolete.

We stayed at the Miramar in the center of downtown Waikiki, among the dozens of other resorts and hotels. We were on the 12th floor, where the four of us crashed in a room with an outside balcony long enough for us to conveniently relax. Our innovative minds told us the balcony was the perfect bunker to observe any *hotties* who chose to lay out on the deck below us. I couldn't help but remember that I brought my binoculars ("binocs," as Jesse liked to call them).

While every aspect of the trip was enjoyable, there were two experiences that elevated me to esoteric states of mind. Surfing was one of them. We rented twelve-foot-long boards for the two days we surfed. The swells were slow rollers and topped out at three feet at Waikiki Beach. My first two attempts were unsuccessful because of inexperience and poor judgment of wave selection. The third time was a charm. I paddled just over a hundred yards from shore, unsure if I could touch bottom. My wave of choice was as big as they got that day, and I was perfectly positioned, rigorously paddling away from the swell. As it closed in, I lifted off my stomach and onto my hands and knees. The wave began to break, lifting me to its peak as I focused on balance and carefully attempted to stand up. Just as the wave proceeded to an optimum momentum, I rose to the occasion. At that moment I understood a surfer's passion. The Beach Boys' lyrics resonated in my head: "Catch a wave and your sittin' on top of the world." The solitude of euphoria carried me nearly the length of a football field as I managed to carve subtle turns on the long board. It was instant cloud 9.

Weeks before departure to Oahu, my good friend Sean Coyle reminded me that he lived in Hawaii for three years. His father was an admiral in the navy. Sean urged us to rent mopeds because it's one of the most raw and cheap ways to explore the island. Upon our second day in Oahu, Mike, Jesse, Dave, and I did exactly that. We rode like we owned the island, carefree, as if we were obnoxious little kids, peeling out on lawns of other residencies, weaving through traffic, and howling like wild animals.

The day before our vacation was over, we had no concrete plans, but one thing we all wanted to do was moped for a second time. Hung over from a booze cruise the night before, we contemplated our routes. Mike was set with riding around the island, Dave was thinking about riding up Diamond Head; Jesse and I weren't too sure, although both options sounded appealing. Conclusively, Jesse and Dave rode up to Diamond Head while Mike and I began our trek around the island.

On a moderately cool day, topping out at thirty-five miles per hour, the island breeze streaked across our faces. I constantly reminded myself to validate the distinction between beauty and the never-ending buzz of the rental moped. Cruising along the North Shore was nothing short of breathtaking. The differentiation of surrounding wilderness and the greenery of the highlands was as distinct and plush as cumulous clouds. The spectacle of rolling swells and crashing waves was a privilege in itself. Along the shoreline, surfers swayed and weaved in their everyday ritual, which I both envied and admired.

Throughout the day, rain sprinkled for short, intermittent intervals, transforming cool into cold and rays of sunshine into sighs of relief. By the time we concluded the journey, we rode well over 100 miles around the perimeter of the island, minus the vicinity of Pearl Harbor. It took us over five hours. Along the way we encountered numerous moments of awe and a few moments of misfortune.

Mike and I alternated the lead throughout our trek. Luckily I brought a jacket and a pair of sunglasses to obstruct the wind and any roaming bugs that might try to fly into my eyes. Mike, on the other hand, wore eyeglasses but fell short of a windbreaker and was drenched most of the time. Throughout various legs of the excursion, I'd lend him my jacket, leaving me face-to-face with the elements. On some stretches rain would soak us like someone turned on a shower. Then, just like that, the rain would completely shut off. The exchange between scenery and enduring the elements gave me a more pure and appreciative perspective of island behavior.

For the second half of the trek, it rained and poured as we became drenched to the bone—not to mention the fact that we were hungry, too. About 20 miles away from making full circle, Mike ran over a nail and blew one of his tires as we rode along the shoulder of an interstate highway. (Not a very good idea when riding up a grade at thirty miles an hour while passing traffic zooms by at sixty-five.) We didn't know our way around, but we knew that scaling the highway would eventually get us back to the Miramar.

It took over an hour between walking the scooter to an off ramp, calling the rental company to report the flat tire, waiting in the rain, and having someone come to replace the entire bike instead of the tire. When we finally got situated, I called our hotel and Dave answered the phone. Both he and Jesse had been relaxing for almost two hours since their excursion up to Diamond Head. Dave laughed hysterically as I explained our misfortune. Fortunately we made it back in time to prepare for dinner with Jesse's relatives.

My most captivating moment of the Hawaiian vacation, however, came at a pineapple stand with Mike. Since we began our journey, we rode nearly two hours until we reached a surmised halfway point, where he suggested we stop at the next pineapple stand. I craved nourishment. Ten minutes later we found ourselves at a tropical fruit stand that sold pineapples, oranges, papayas, coconuts, bananas, and a variety of nuts. The price was two dollars per pineapple, so we split the cost. The merchant informed us of two different types of pineapple taste: tart and sweet or tangy and tart. We decided to go with tart and sweet.

The mood mysteriously changed at the moment of purchase. The clouds dispersed, allowing the sun to radiate and warm us. After we sat on a bench next to our mopeds, Mike pulled out a small pocketknife. The blade wasn't long enough to make one clean slice, so we alternated to cut our own chunks. Juice secreted from every incision as if we squeezed a wet sponge. The juice was like syrup. As Rob Schneider from *Saturday Night Live* would say, "You lika dey juice, eh? Dey juice is good. I get you some juice." I lika dey juice!

My taste buds orgasmed as I sunk my teeth into the first chunk; it was like eating the nectar of the gods or some type of forbidden fruit. I lost count of how many times I repeated, "This is sssooooooo good" after I said it twice. I *mmmm*'ed and *ahhhh*'d. Mike indulged as much as I did but was more passive about his commentary. He just seemed to nod his head after each of my remarks. Our fingers glazed with pineapple juice as we slowly devoured quite possibly the best pineapple in the world.

A tour bus pulled to the side of the road where Mike and I were gorging. My cheeks and hands were layered with pineapple juice as if I were an infant learning to eat. I remember the observation from the people on the bus. They must have thought we were cavemen. Out of nowhere, Mike nodded his head again and humbly stated, "Now this is living!"

A DAY FROZEN IN TIME – MONDAY, MAY 17

Once again I wake up with the same familiar discomfort. This time it's worse than ever. My daily updates and consistent symptoms keep my dad well informed on my situation. Currently, Europe is scheduled to begin within the next 30 hours, and at this point there is a stamp on my agenda that says, "URGENT." My dad and I agreed to take me down to the ER at Saint Mary's Hospital to be evaluated. After checking in, filling out paperwork, and getting clearance on insurance, I awaited my fate.

The wait wasn't too long for someone to call my name for evaluation. Following an initial series of questions, I was escorted to a room full of small machines and medical equipment. Soon, other hospital staff inquired about my status. A curtain dangled down at the halfway point in the room to separate any awkward stares between myself and another potentially traumatized patient. I did not yet know that I was the one traumatized. A nurse directed me to sit in an optometrist patient's high-back chair, where I would wait another few minutes until someone finally tended to me. Soon, doctors and nurses asked me questions to lay a foundation, and my verbal responses summoned curiosity. The next thing I know they're insisting on putting an IV catheter into my wrist. "Go ahead," I thought and agreed. After all, I just wanted to go to Europe.

I became numb and drowsy within seconds after an unknown anesthetic drug was injected into my IV. The sedative nearly put me to sleep. While escorted and randomly tested in various unknown areas of the hospital over a two-hour period, I experienced my first chest X-ray and CT scan. My curiosity and awareness of the oddity of events transpiring was blinded by the excitement to reach Europe. I could've cared less about anything as long as I was in Bilbao, Spain, in the next two days.

After this unusual sequence of events, I ended up in the same room I started. As I sat there in a daze, I noticed my dad talking to a doctor down the hall. I figured he may be getting worried because it had been over two hours since I left him in the waiting room. I concluded my dad wasn't talking to someone about the wait but something far more devastating. To this point I was still clueless. The doctors insisted that I sit in a wheelchair in order to be escorted to him down the hall. "OK," I sarcastically thought to myself. When I reached him, I looked him in the eyes with the "So, what's up?" attitude. He looked very grim, his face frozen like stone as if he just saw Medusa.

"It doesn't look like you're going to Europe," he said. "The doctors think you may have a tumor." And just like that . . .

KABOOOOOOOOOOOOOOM. There went the neighborhood.

I was shocked and speechless. My life was instantaneously engaged into surreal, super-slow motion with a numbness that paralyzed my psyche. I don't know if I was so overwhelmed by the initial impact of the bad news, but the first thing that came to my mind was, "There goes Europe." Other than graduation and the holidays, I don't remember when the last time my dad outright gave me a hug based on an occasion other than special. This wasn't a special occasion but a true mark of unconditional love and support. I didn't know what to feel or how to feel as my face remained unexpressive. Shocked, for lack of a better word. Evidently the news reached my mother before me because she was already on her way to the hospital.

Minutes after the devastating news, the doctors put me on a stretcher to be wheeled to another room. As a nurse pushed me down a hallway, I noticed my mom just feet away. I demanded the nurse to stop as I began to reach out for my mother. At this moment I realized that the impact of recent events didn't really affect me until I saw the impact it made on her. The look on her face was a mirror image of what my dad and I were feeling—shocked and overwhelmed. Paralyzed in disbelief, I resorted to being strong, but the force of the conviction and the looks on Mom's and Dad's faces were too mighty for me to bear. My eyes welled up as tears instantly streamed down my face. We embraced each other tightly.

After the first episode of emotions, I was escorted further down the hall, where the doctors and nurses transferred me to a one-bed hospital room. I was given an anti-seizure drug called Dilantin and a steroid called Decadron. Decadron was intended to relieve edema (swelling) in my head. I was told to basically strip and put on a hospital gown. So I did, unsure if I was living in denial or reality. I then decided to lie on a bed while infinite thoughts aimlessly. It didn't take long for me to make a cry for help to anyone that I considered a friend. I picked up the phone at my bedside. Meanwhile, Mom and Dad were informing my family graduation spectators over a different phone. Everyone except for Aunt Sherre, Aunt Betty, and Uncle Marvin were on their way home. They were in as much disbelief as anyone else who knew me.

Through these initial moments things were going in slow motion—I suppose like being burned alive. The only things I could think of to douse the flames were my friends. I knew if I waited too long to find salvation, I would be badly scared from loneliness. From this moment through the next three days, the images and faces of the people who would be there to support me remain branded in my memory.

There are times in life when certain things are highlighted more than others. During this experience there were countless highlighted moments, both high and low. I do remember the first significant moment in particular. The first person I called was one of my best friends, Mark Wood. Mark and I became friends our sophomore year in high school, when we *made* the junior varsity baseball team as underdogs. Over recent summers we played golf and tennis every week, and it just so happened that he was at home when I called to break the news. He couldn't believe it. With no hesitation he was at the hospital in minutes. Prior to his arrival, I called other close friends.

When Mark arrived, I was lying on my hospital bed. We shook hands as he took a seat. His eyes became red as he tried to fight off the welling tears. The whole situation was "bullshit," as he would say, and it was. Judging by the look on his face, I think he was more shaken up than I was at the time. I was at comfort with him being there, while he was still absorbing the shock. Inside I was still numb but not shattered as I told him more on the predicament as optimistically as possible. He comprehended with reassurance that things would be fine. Mark was the catalyst who reassured me that he would be one of the many people that I could always rely on for unconditional friendship and support.

My main frustration stemmed from the fact that my aspiration to back-pack Europe was now crippled by a faceless enemy. Chris Crawforth, my longtime friend since T-ball, was my would-be travel compadre to Europe and was obviously among the first people I called after diagnosis. Chris and I had known each other since we were teammates in Little League. After a night of sleeping on it, Chris did what I would have done: he went to Europe. Europe was like a graduation present to ourselves because we knew that, if we didn't do it now, it could be a while before, if ever, we had a chance to go again. My time would come, we agreed.

At first sight or first notice, I'm sure everybody who came to visit me went through some form of shock, but I didn't feel sorry for myself nor did it seem apparent in anyone else. Before diagnosis I was very much driven and in control of my life, and it would take more than a brain tumor to keep me down. As time slowly strolled by, friends would pass in and out of my hospital room. Awkward, but mainly out of concern and curiosity, they would ask the obvious, "how?" or "why?" I was as uneducated about cancer and tumors as most anyone at age 23. My reply was, "I have a brain infection that may be a tumor. It is the size of a golf ball and needs to be removed ASAP."

The brief, formatted conversations were all similar. Many asked questions such as, "Do they [the doctors] know how you may have gotten it?"

"I don't know, but after they take out the tumor, they will do tests on the tissue and we'll find out," I replied, as if I was right.

"How did you know something was wrong?"

"I had these really bad headaches for the past week and a half. When I woke up this morning, they were worse than ever, so my dad took me to the hospital. The doctors took a CT scan, a chest X-ray, and concluded that I had a brain tumor."

One doctor told me, "The tumor may have been growing two or three years ago, but you didn't have any clinical symptoms until last week. It's tough to say. It may have started to grow in recent months."

One of my fraternity pledge brothers, Chris LaRose, told me of his mother who had a tumor in her lung. "She's doing great," he said. I felt some comfort when Chris shared his mom's story with me. Dustin Reed, another one of my pledge brothers, was there with his future wife, Amanda. They were dating at the time. Amanda shared with me that her mother once had a stroke. What I can remember best about it was that her mom's memory wasn't as good as it once was, and she got tired real easily. She was a survivor, which was all that really mattered to me.

I was told by a doctor that tumors have no distinct diagnosis regarding why and how they form, although there are reasonable possibilities. One could say that they're inherited mutations or hormone dysfunctions. The list can be long and technical; but call it what you will: a tumor is a tumor, and it sucks. I wasn't too concerned about researching the cause because, quite frankly, I had to deal with the present. My intention was to overcome it and get on with my life.

CHAPTER 2

LIGHTNING CRASHES

TUESDAY – MAY 18, 1999

In general, no news is good news, but in my case, the news was bad for everyone. I contacted my closest friends, and the response snowballed. From the next few hours to the next few days, word spread around college campus as several dozen people came to support me. Along with my family, they were my alliance of the war declared . . . my motivation . . . my hope. Those whom I grew up with—unconditional friends from the beginning, fraternity brothers, Mom's church friends, engineering friends from school, and other caring acquaintances—I was deeply humbled with their overwhelming support and attention. The gathering lifted me onto a pedestal of courage and confidence.

I learned that the unconditional response of "being there" can mean the world. Those who came to support me were a great distraction, and words can't express my gratitude of those whom were there. The thought that I might have cancer seemed inconceivable, especially fresh out of college. A new foundation was being built beneath me, one that would become a temple of hope. Most of the time I was entertained by sharing sarcasm and laughter with anyone who walked into my room. It was the support of these friends that gave me hope and helped sustain my sanity. Surgery was expected to take place on Thursday.

WEDNESDAY - MAY 19

My hospital room became a thing of beauty. Dozens of floral arrangements decorated the windowsill, along with several dozen get-well cards. My dad knew how important music was to me, and he bought a boom box along with a handful of CDs I requested from home to help the time pass in my hospital room.

After the last of my friends went home on the eve of my operation, things started to quiet down, and the ever-so-harsh reality of what I was about to face began to set in. All I could do was hold on and hope that the tides would not sweep me away. A true warrior might say that one must accept the fact that a war has been declared. To be a leader in this battle, it would be up to me to direct my army to defeat the adversary.

Through college I've learned it's best to live in the moment and, if possible, avoid jumping to any conclusions, although a lot of times it's hard to keep anxiety at bay. Either out of all honesty or total ignorance, I was only afraid of brain surgery. I believed that my tumor was just a bump in the road, no pun intended, and within a couple months I'd be on with my life. Nobody told me I had cancer, nor was it proven. In fact I didn't even consider it.

One of the hardest things to swallow, however, was that the reality I was now living didn't seem possible. So young, healthy, and energetic, it was a shock for anyone to see me in this state of turmoil. From personal experience I testify that, when something like this happens, its tough to keep your emotions in check. All kinds of crazy thoughts arose in my head throughout the past three days. What I knew about tumors at the time was that they were either cancerous or had the potential to be cancerous. Brain surgery? I mean, like, come on. Cynically speaking, I thought brain surgery was the type of thing that only existed in those black-and-white Frankenstein movies, like the one where the mad scientist switches a monkey brain to a human body. *Who or what would I become?*

A DAY NOT WELL REMEMBERED - THURSDAY, MAY 20

As far as I can recall, I was awakened at 6:00 a.m. when a nurse promptly guided me onto a stretcher and rolled me to the prep room for surgery. Upon arrival, I became acutely aware that I was not the only patient in the room. I was on my back, rolling my head from side to side to see who else occupied the area. There were at least three other patients who looked just as lost as I was, but what their diagnosis or prognosis was seemed totally irrelevant. My parents and other random doctors and nurses also occupied the room.

Following the majority of the preparation for surgery, I was given "happy medicine," an anesthetic drug that would help me relax and think lightly. I felt a little loony in a carefree, stoned fashion. Before the anesthesia could take its full effect, I remember hugging Mom and Dad, and my dad said, "See you on the other side." Mom said, "I love you." The last thing I remembered was being wheeled to the operating room for surgery and the removal of my tumor. I don't know how, but if I died during surgery, I would die painlessly, in my sleep.

I felt like the victim in a science fiction movie. You know, the one where someone gets abducted by aliens and is pulled into the alien mother ship by a beam of light. I had no control over the alien power, and the alien beings could do whatever they wanted to me. I was forced into a state of denial because fear would consume me more than I could control. And so the surgery took place . . .

After surgery, I vaguely remember a few episodes. The room was bright with an ample aura of hospital lights. I woke up breathing heavily, and I was terrified. My body's natural response from the anesthesia to consciousness was quicker than normal; however it was a good sign that I was healthy and alert. I was alive! During the time of my awakening, I vaguely remember talking to my parents and receiving smiles of reassurance. I remember talking to my friend Paul Sifre and receiving similar support. Paul worked at the hospital at the time. Other than that, the next episode I remembered was waking up alone in a dark, desolate, intensive-care room.

FRIDAY – MAY 21

How in the hell did I move from point A to point B? It felt as if I just woke up from a nightmare. Or was I still in the nightmare? I felt very confused and different. I had no idea what had happened, what day it was, and, for a moment, where I was. *What year is it, and am I still me?* It was as if I had just awakened from a long, deep coma, my body drained and senseless. I later learned the real story of a two-day block of my life that never seemed to exist. So, what really happened, and why was everything so jacked up? A few weeks later, my mom filled me in on the details.

Evidently I was doing just fine after the craniotomy. I began to wake up from the anesthesia around 2 p.m. I was talking, smiling, and even cracking jokes. Things went well throughout the day as I slowly began to recover in an intensive-care unit. Around six o'clock the next morning, I was talking to my neurosurgeon, Dr. John Davis, a nurse, and my parents. Suddenly I passed out, had a seizure, and didn't wake up. Dr. Davis cleared everyone from the room, and I was rushed to the emergency room to undergo a second craniotomy. With other assistance, Dr. Davis opened my skull for a second time and began to operate. He removed more dead tissue in addition to what was taken out from the first surgery, which was a mass the size of a racquetball.

From the supposed initial infection, the seizure was caused by additional brain swelling. The swelling is the reason I felt pressure in my head, which landed me in the hospital in the first place. For precaution and prevention of more seizures, my original skull flap was temporarily removed. Would I ever have a full, natural cranium again? I did not know. Unless I wore a helmet, there would be no acceptable form of protection if I took a fall except for the flesh covering my brain.

When I had a sense of cognition after I awakened from the second operation, reality seemed surreal. The visual atmosphere was the complete opposite from my awakening of the first surgery. It was dark, I was alone, and instead of smiles and laughter, there was a haunting silence assisted by the beeping of my heart monitor. I could sense voices and the reverberation of footsteps walking up and down the hall. I thought to myself, *"What . . . the hell . . . is going on?"*

I noticed many discouraging elements as I tried to orient myself. I was totally discombobulated and very weak physically. I could barely talk to myself without slurring words. I felt like a rag doll that had been beaten with an ugly stick. At least I knew who I was. Slowly I began to realize the damage done. When I began to acknowledge myself, I slowly reached up to touch the top of my head. Although my dome was wrapped in bandages, I could feel a hollow spot. There was an indent where the surgery took place. I was cautious as hell when I felt my new contours. I couldn't believe it, and what the hell was this plastic breathing thing in my nose? My line of sight was extremely distorted and obnoxious, but that was only a small part of my large problem.

I began to explore the new tubes and other accessories that had either been connected to, or were already inserted into, my body. One of the first things I noticed was the massage pads that were wrapped around each leg from thigh to ankle. About every minute or two the pads would lightly squeeze my legs and decompress. They were used to help prevent blood clots. Fair enough. There was a breathing apparatus in my nose. There were IV's in both of my arms. Great. Not only was I missing a chunk of my skull and a part of my brain, but I was also a human pincushion.

I noticed a slight discomfort around my groin area. I reached down carefully, and to my dismay I noticed a catheter was buried in my *dick*. At the moment I had no idea what it was or what it was used for; the catheter, that is. Being in my groin and all, I immediately asked the nurse what it was. She told me it was a Foley catheter, used to keep a constant measurement of my urine and to control my bladder. Obviously it had to be taken out.

While I was lying in bed, concerned friends continued to visit me. In most cases, guests would be prohibited after an operation such as mine. My mom, dad, and recent hospital staff knew how much the support meant to me. My room was the party of the hospital, and an exception was made for anyone who desired to visit. The first to visit while I lay lifeless were two of my engineering peers with whom I graduated only six days ago: Dan and Daigo. I was grumpy as hell, barely mobile. I snapped at both and slurred slowly, "What the hell are you doing here . . . Get out of here . . . You shouldn't be here." They looked shocked and concerned. I don't know what surprised them the most, my condition or my attitude. Probably both. They slowly backed away and walked out the door. I felt bad because they were there to support me, and all I could do was drive them away. Perhaps I was still in a state of shock and didn't know how to react. I shed a tear and thought to myself, "I can't believe I just did that."

The next guest to arrive was over an hour later. It was my friend Erick Wipf, one of my party buddies. He sat in a chair across the room as we spoke nonsense about whatever it was we talked about while I struggled to mumble my comments. I guess it was raining and storming outside, so we talked about the wind and lightning. I don't remember the details, but I do remember laughing about stupid stuff and sharing obnoxious noises, like "Ehhhh" and "Eee."

PRELUDE TO RELEASE - MAY 22-MAY 30

After four days in intensive care, the catheter in my groin became way too bothersome. With a little whining and puppy-dog eyes, I convinced my nurse to have it removed. I became very nervous and uncomfortable. The nurse said it wouldn't be that bad. Boy was she wrong. First she measured then emptied the rest of my urine into the toilet. When she came back I grew nervous with every breath. "On the count of three," she said, One, two . . ." *Three* was when I felt the life being sucked out of me as the catheter was pulled out. I intended to watch but the second I felt the pulling I couldn't help but yelp and cringe. I didn't bother to look after it was removed. They end up being four or five inches long while three of those inches was buried in my bladder. I couldn't move for about a minute because of the incredible discomfort. I was stunned.

During the seizure a pupil was blown in my left eye due to the excess swelling of my brain. My line of sight with both eyes was no longer horizontal. With either eye closed and the other one open, things appeared normal.

With both eyes open there was a distinct error. As my dad described it: "The images overlapped each other on a vertical axis." Days later, the doctors gave me an eye patch so I could focus on things one eye at a time. I didn't care what I looked like, I just wanted to go home.

Nick Stolpman, a close friend of mine since our junior year in high school, revisited me one day. My mom prepared fresh homemade burritos for both of us. She arranged them with fresh lettuce and tomato on the side. Since we became friends in high school, Nick has always been helpless when it comes to Mom's burritos. He was feeling satisfied with one, while I preferred to continue eating until I could go no longer. It was a great escape from the bland hospital food.

Upon my request the CT scan was revealed to me. I knew that the tumor was the size of a golf ball, but I never had the chance to see it until now. With contrast the film highlighted the affected areas of the tumor. My tumor looked like a nebula. I was prescribed a temporary low dose of Decadron to assist in the reduction of any swelling of the brain after a craniotomy. Dilantin was still prescribed to reduce chances of seizures.

During the last few days at St. Mary's, I slowly began to regain a sense of self and control. Friends showed up daily to express concern and to make me laugh and reminisce. Doctors and nurses educated me on the various complications I was going to face, such as short-term memory loss and trouble with speech and constructive thinking. To keep up a fight and try to stay mentally focused, I had to be as strong-willed as possible. For the time being, my first objective was to get out of the hospital and back into a cozy home.

CHAPTER 3

EYE OF THE VORTEX

According to the original game plan, Eurail was supposed to be my main method of transit, while accommodations were provided in youth hostels. Instead I spent recent weeks on gurneys and wheelchairs to transport me in a hospital. I should have been having the time of my life, backpacking in Europe. The plan was to begin in Spain, Eurail through France, hang out in Italy for at least a week, hit Switzerland for a couple days, and on to Germany, where Chris and I would rendezvous with our childhood friend Jeff Dawson. By now my trek with Chris would be somewhere in either Switzerland or Germany.

The cumulative stint at St. Mary's Regional Medical Center lasted exactly two weeks: three days preparing, two days in surgery, six days recovering in intensive care, and another few days to gain enough strength so I could be sent home. Personally, I felt healthy enough to leave days before my actual release. Those final days in the hospital seemed unnecessary and hindered my progress to well being. In retrospect I truly think my stay could have been two days less. My release was on Monday, May 30, and it never felt so good to be home.

Like the aftermath of a tornado, my cognitive mind was scattered and distorted. At first I really couldn't do anything effectively. I couldn't remember names or experiences that I would have otherwise boasted about. Sometimes I slurred my words, and most of the time I couldn't complete a narrative thought. I was constantly at a loss for words.

I had tremendous difficulty with handwriting and typing. I once became so frustrated while writing a check that I broke down in tears. No matter how hard I tried, my neurons wouldn't allow me to put my thoughts down on paper. Legible print became scribbles.

Responding and explaining was another obvious setback in my intellect. It seemed my IQ had been reduced to that of a kindergartener. I was told by the doctors and rehab counselors that the brain has a natural way of repairing itself. Hopefully my neurons would agree because for the time being my short-term memory was in ruins.

My situation was considered a medical emergency. Things moved so fast in the first two weeks that no one had a chance to conclude with a what, why, and how I came up with this problem. Lab work and studies were done at an urgent rate from the moment I was diagnosed with a brain tumor. At this stage the tumor wasn't yet proven to be benign or malignant.

LABORATORY DATA: RADIOLOGICAL STUDIES WHICH WERE REVIEWED INCLUDED A BRAIN MRI SCAN DONE ON 6-16-99, WHICH REVEALED SLIGHTLY INCREASED ENHANCEMENT WITHIN THE RESIDUAL LEFT PARIENTAL TUMOR, COMPARED WITH THE PATIENT'S IMMEDIATE POSTOPERATIVE SCAN OF 5-25-99. THE LESION COMES UP TO THE CORTICAL SURFACE AND IS APPROXIMATELY 4 CM X 4 CM.

Originally my case was forwarded to a tumor board at the University of California, San Francisco. There, a conclusive surgery and diagnosis was meant to take place after final pathology reports were determined. Doctors of St. Mary's and UCSF worked together on my case, but neither could confirm a diagnosis. Biopsy samples were taken from my tissue blocks to see if the cultures would grow, yet I never heard of any progress firsthand. The word *lymphoma* popped up every now and then, but there was never a final verdict. For one, I didn't know what lymphoma was, nor did I ever ponder the fact that I might have cancer. I thought lymphoma was lymphoma, not a form of cancer; it certainly didn't sound threatening. My state of denial kept me sane and optimistic during this time. Other general assumptions were leukemia, multiple sclerosis, HIV, and meningitis. "Every possibility needs to be checked," said one nurse. At this point of progress, all results were negative, although lymphoma was the presumed original diagnosis from the start.

Needless to say, life was difficult for my family and me because we didn't have the slightest bit of education pertaining to brain tumors. It seemed as if we were marionettes going through the motions.

To make a long story short, UCSF did not have a network doctor who coordinated with my insurance, so my case was sent to UCLA. (Or so it was said.) Six long weeks after my surgeries at St. Mary's, I would wait and wait some more before I would be able to proceed into a final operation. I don't know what the holdup was, but I wanted a clean bill of health so I could get on with my life. One thing was obvious: a final craniotomy would be required before I could even think about moving forward. I wasn't agreeable to that, but there was no protection beyond the extent of my flesh to provide a barrier where a chunk of my skull once was. However, with all the repairing that had been done so far, I knew I was fixable. How much fixable was still the question that only time would tell.

A month of memory and speech therapy convinced me that I was capable of thinking cognitively, only on a much slower and lower scale. Since my line of sight was distorted, I was given an eye patch to concentrate with one eye at a time. Every few hours I would switch to the opposite eye, which was supposed to slowly correct the overlapping error. I felt like the *Goonie* named One-Eyed Willy.

Shortly after I was released from St. Mary's, my vision problems were reduced with a pair of prescription prism lenses. The lenses fit over my regular glasses and were barely noticeable. I wasn't allowed to drive without them. Things were obviously expected to take time. In the meantime I was more occupied with working toward a better state of well being.

MAKING THE BEST OF THINGS
When the dust began to settle from the first two craniotomies, I saw life

from a new perspective. The road ahead was unknown and unmapped, but hope and support from my friends and family granted me the courage to tread the path.

Two weeks before college graduation I was in complete control of my life. Two weeks later I didn't know who I was or where I was going. I was like a dismantled jigsaw puzzle with memories scattered upside-down and portions partially assembled. Certain sections displayed an obvious image, while other pieces didn't seem to fit anywhere. Some couldn't be found at all. It was difficult to link one thought to the next. Granted, I could think with distorted thoughts, but I couldn't communicate effectively.

I pondered and shared questions with certain close friends that would never be answered. It's strange that I was diagnosed the day after my college graduation. Fate or coincidence? What if I had been in Europe, as originally planned, where I hardly knew anyone and this happened? Who knows what kind of medical attention and resources I would have had access to? If the tumor went untreated, how much longer would I live? My health insurance policy, under my mom's name, expired the day I graduated. Luckily my case was an exception to the rule. The insurance that recently expired rolled onto a COBRA plan with the same full medical benefits. Otherwise I was screwed. The difference was a monthly premium, which was nothing compared to the $65,000 medical bill.

As I waited weeks for a phone call with the results of my craniotomy, I tried to make the best of things. The remedy to my inner and neurological struggles was my friends and family. Any time I surrounded myself with them, a blanket of reassurance and safety would soothe my fidgety mental balance—similar to tossing bed sheets over my head when I was a kid. As long as my body and head were covered, the bogeyman couldn't get me. As I was being consumed in the midst of the toughest challenge of my life, I realized that I was backed by the best people in the world. Every phone call or visitation from a friend meant the world to me.

I had distorted vision, balance problems, memory problems, and a hole in my head. After doing the math, the sum total of my thoughts told me to take it easy for a while, but I couldn't sit still. The restlessness of my neurons were seeking a place to channel themselves. I had to put them to work.

A week after my release from St. Mary's, my dad and I went to the library, where he recommended *The Old Man and the Sea* by Ernest Hemingway. All of my mental and physical flaws were painfully relevant as I slowly began to tread through an otherwise easy task. I wondered if I could retain anything. First of all, I was reading with one eye at a time. Without the patch my ability to read was an unpleasant, dizzying task. Nonetheless I progressed through the book in a very slow fashion, concentrating on each sentence, pronouncing multisyllable words like a Hooked on Phonics student. But after two weeks I succeeded with the assignment. To my surprise and enlightenment I comprehended a great majority of the book. It was my first proactive accomplishment. A day or two later I checked out another Hemingway book titled *The Dangerous Summer* and read it in less than three weeks.

After reading a couple of Ernest Hemingway books, writing seemed like an occupation I would rather pursue. What better way to live life than travel the world and write? Reading outweighed a lot of my frustrations. It was something inanimate yet mind stimulating. The next book I began to read was one recommended by a dear friend, Jennifer Enos. She let me borrow *The Celestine Prophecy* by James Redfield, and it couldn't have arrived at a better time.

Redfield described the journey in his book as a series of insights, coincidences, and intuitions. Similar to what I was going through, I found peace within my friends, my family, literature, music, and within myself—the best things in life. Through all the medical trauma it was as if I was learning about these things for the very first time and I couldn't ignore them. There somehow seemed to be an underlying master plan that I did not yet understand. But the writing on the wall, The Beatles and the Dave Matthews Band, said it all when they sang, "All you need is love" and "Love is all you need."

Aside from reading, I pursued a more demanding chore: music. I love music. For nine years I endured piano lessons, beginning when I was eight years old. I knew a variety of songs from memory, but after my heinous operation I couldn't recall anything. The same had to do with playing the guitar, which I taught myself in college. Finger coordination and muscle memory were far from par, and I couldn't play short, simple riffs. Heck, I couldn't even remember them. The dexterity in my hands was traumatized and awkward. It was as if I never picked up a guitar in my entire life.

I'd periodically attempt to play one or the other, and they merged into a very frustrating learning curve. I had to retrain my hand-eye coordination, and the more my hands were on the instruments, the more I recalled. It was as if I reached an epiphany every week. On a scale of 1 to 10, my progress was about 2.5 by my next craniotomy. Picking up my guitar or touching the keys on the piano was a form of salvation, no matter how arduous or flawed.

Between craniotomies my greatest feeling of life emanated from the beaches of Lake Tahoe. It's arguably the most beautiful natural lake in the world and humbling to anyone who takes a glance at it. I remember many great times camping, backpacking, mountain biking, partying, and beach bumming. There was nothing more to ask for than 90-degree weather while sunbathing under a cloudless sky with close friends and beautiful women. During the weeks between operations, the three times I was at Lake Tahoe elevated me to the purest sensation of life. Tahoe is so serene and peaceful that it's easy to lose yourself into thinking about anything or nothing at all. I chose the latter.

BACK TO THE LECTURE AT HAND - JULY 2

Tomorrow couldn't arrive soon enough. The obstacle of anxiety was poignant, and time would soon tap on my shoulder to tell me to move forward. The only sure thing was that another surgery would be required for a prolonged, natural, normal life at best.

FINDINGS: IN THE INTERVAL, THERE HAS BEEN RESECTION OF A LARGE TUMOR IN THE LEFT PARIENTAL LOBE. ON THE POST CONTRAST IMAGES, THICK IRREGULAR ENHANCEMENT IS SEEN IN THE ANTERIOR INFERIOR MARGIN OF THE RESECTION CAVITY REPRESENTING RESIDUAL TUMOR. MILD MASS EFFECT IS STILL SEEN, SECONDARY TO THE LEFT CEREBRAL EDEMA. THE RESIDUAL EDEMA IS MODERATE IN DEGREE AND IT EXTENDS TO THE MARGIN OF THE ATRIUM OF THE LEFT LATERAL VENTRICAL.

My post craniotomy scar was well healed but still moderately sunken because I had no bone flap over the previous wound. Hearing was slightly decreased in my left ear to whispers and finger rubs. All other cardiovascular functions were normal.

When all bureaucratic issues were resolved through UCSF, my case was forwarded to UCLA Medical Center. The powers that be finally gave me the opportunity to continue with a consultation on Friday, July 8, at UCLA.

JULY 3-7

My dad was born and raised in Southern California. As soon as we found out our next chess move, we flew to Los Angeles, where we visited and stayed with various branches of family. Our primary intention was to meet the active hospital staff involved with my case. Plus, it was a relief to get out of town. Because of work constraints my mom stayed in Reno, barring any major events that may have caused her to come down. It was tough.

My dad and I stayed with The Munseys, a close family branch on my dad's side. Aunt Joan found success in real estate, Uncle Ray was a fire chief, Cousin Scott was a surfer, Cousin Julie and husband Stacy were expecting, and Cousin Christine was attending college at UCSB. Joan and Ray's home was a great sanctuary to escape and relieve some anxiety. They owned a house that was part of a lake community. When you walked out the back door, there was a dock and a patio. It was so relaxing to take a ride, and I fell in love with the place. In fact, I told my dad, "This is the type of lifestyle I want to live."

Dad and I rented a car, which enabled us to also visit Aunt Dorothy, Uncle Carl, Aunt Lucy, and Uncle Glen. My Aunt Melva lived two blocks away from the beach in Santa Monica. We also drove along parts of the coast, and he showed me where he used to hang as a kid, including Santa Monica pier, Zuma Beach, and Malibu Beach.

On July 4 my dad and I decided to see the Dodgers play the Giants. The Giants prevailed, and after the game a lengthy fireworks show took place. It was a special time for us to enjoy something we both loved as kids.

JULY 8

We met my new neurosurgeon, Dr. Linda Liau, who was very clear and concise as she answered our questions and concerns. Her confidence and kind demeanor seduced my trust within the first few minutes of our meeting. At the consultation my dad and I were given the opportunity to sit down and listen to what was involved in the procedure. Our questions were answered, and our concerns were expressed.

Our checklist was long, but nobody was going anywhere. We needed every bit of information before any drastic decisions were made for a final surgery. One of our first intuitions regarded my MRI and CT scans, which showed where the tumor roughly originated and where dead tissue had already been taken out. We were told that there was no sign of tumor growth on the current MRI since the first resections.

The tumor originated on the front left side of my brain where it grew over time. For how long and how fast, nobody really knew, but based on its size, other doctors assumed it may have started growing a few years earlier. The MRI scans gave me a better illustration of what my brain once looked like before surgery. More than half of what was removed during the surgeries was larger than a golf ball. It was clearly evident that I went through an extreme experience. According to an article I read in a publication from

Memorial Sloan-Kettering Cancer Center, it can take up to thirty years for a tumor to develop and become large enough to produce clinical symptoms. I didn't experience severe, consistent symptoms until twelve days before I had it removed. I was only twenty-three.

Dr. John Davis in Reno removed the bulk of the tumor. Because there hadn't been a conclusive diagnosis at the time, he was well aware that he couldn't remove it all. There was a definite risk that I would lose motor skills, specifically speech. The remaining part of the tumor had grown into the speech and language part of my brain. It was Dr. Linda Liau's job to clean up any residual tissue left from the earlier operations to ensure the best possible outcome without infiltrating my motor senses.

> **ASSESSMENT & PLAN:** THIS IS A 23-YEAR-OLD RIGHT HANDED YOUNG MAN APPROXIMATELY SIX WEEKS STATUS POST A SUBTOTAL RESECTION OF A LEFT PARIENTAL TUMOR AT AN OUTSIDE HOSPITAL. THE DIAGNOSIS AT THIS POINT, WHEN REVIEWED BY UCSF, REVEALED THAT THE PATIENT'S DIAGNOSIS WAS MOST LIKELY A LYMPHOMA, PER OUTSIDE PATHOLOGY. HOWEVER, THE SLIDES ARE CURRENTLY BEING REVIEWED HERE AT UCLA NEUROPATHOLOGY TO CONFIRM THIS DIAGNOSIS. HIS FOLLOW-UP MRI SCAN DONE HERE AT UCLA 6-16-99 REVEALS AN INTERVAL INCREASE IN THE CONTRAST ENHANCING LESION IN THE LEFT PARIENTAL AREA, CONSISTENT WITH POSSIBLE PROGRESSION OF DISEASE AND CAUSING SIGNIFICANT MASS EFFECT AND EDEMA.
>
> GIVEN THE RAPID INTERVAL CHANGE IN THE PATIENT'S LEFT PARIETAL RESIDUAL LESION AND THE UNCLEAR PATHOLOGICAL DIAGNOSIS, IT WAS FELT THAT THE PATIENT SHOULD UNDERGO REPEAT RESECTION OF HIS TUMOR FOR DEBULKING AND DEFINITIVE DIAGNOSIS. THE PATIENT WILL ALSO UNDERGO CRANIOPLASTY WITH TITANIUM MESH

AND PONE SOURCE AT THE TIME OF SURGERY TO CORRECT
HIS CRANIAL DEFECT. THE PROCEDURE ALONG WITH ITS
INDICATIONS, RISKS AND POSSIBLE COMPLICATIONS WERE ALL
EXPLAINED IN DETAIL TO THE PATIENT AND HIS FATHER. THEY
UNDERSTOOD AND AGREED TO PROCEED WITH SURGERY 7-19-99.

LINDA LIAU, M.D.
CC: TIMOTHY CLOUGHESY, M.D.

Just like my dad later told other close relatives, "They took out a piece of
his skull the size of a baseball card." The next question of interest was, what
was going to compensate for the portion of my skull that was removed after
the first two craniotomies? There were two options. The first was to have a
premade mold of my head of near perfect contours. That meant I would have
to wait at least another week before the operation. Another week to get the
show on the road was too long for me; besides I wasn't concerned about cos-
metics or prosthetics.

The second option was to have Dr. Liau mold the new cranium with
her own hands as a final task toward completing my operation. This method
would also be the most natural solution in the long run. It's only downside
was the chance of an abnormality in the shape of my head. I gambled with
option two. A synthetic, titanium type of solution would be made for the
new dome. The plate would be held to my head with small titanium screws.
According to its chemistry, the plate is harder than bone, it wouldn't set
off metal detectors, and my hair would grow back. I doubted that it would
attract lightning, but the odds seemed somewhat probable. Stricken with a
brain tumor, electrocuted by lightning, same difference.

Weighing the risks and evaluating other options than surgery was
another complicated process. Although deep down I knew surgery was the
best and most obvious solution, the decision was still difficult, even after
analyzing the short-term and long-term outlooks. The whole concept of

brain surgery left me with an anything-goes attitude. A very ignorant short-term solution would be to forget the surgery, do an alternative treatment, and live life in a world of uncertainty. Who knew what radiation and chemotherapy would do if my tumor was proven to be cancer; at the time I sure as hell didn't. My resistance to contemplate was the only obstruction that separated me from the temptation of becoming miserable.

The final major decision to be made was *my* final decision. It was the toughest, although deep down I knew it was the right one, the only one I could make. I had faith in Dr. Liau because she opened me to confront the probabilities face-to-face. The conflict between fear and hope in my final decision was probably the most difficult. The risks involved waged a major battle within me of optimism and uncertainty. My hope was to recover for a couple months and get on with my life and hopefully still fulfill my graduation trip to Europe.

According to my thoughts between the first and last operations, I really didn't have any intense feelings for living or dying. I was still traumatized like a zombie stuck between two worlds. I couldn't find purpose or meaning that related to my situation, let alone not knowing anyone who had remotely come close to experiencing what was happening to me. The only thing I knew for sure was, if I was to come out of this alive, I would have to survive the third craniotomy; then perhaps I could live in a world where the grass is greener. Until then, nothing was guaranteed.

My journey through life was deeply spiritual and surreal. I didn't know if I would triumph over my condition or live my life as a vegetable. I would have to beat the odds no matter how ordinary or extreme, as the third craniotomy date was scheduled for July 19.

There are risks in surgeries such as this. Like any other challenge in life, there are always risks that could lead to success or failure. Some are of greater magnitude than others. The possibilities range from manageable side effects to minor mental problems, stroke, or even death. Failure could not be an option. The decision was in my hands to weigh and finalize. I chose hope.

CHAPTER 4

SURVIVING THE WAKE

Meanwhile, outside of my traumatized little world, there were two people stronger than I would ever have to be: Mom and Dad. I am an only child. Ted and Kim Heinsohn raised me and have supported me in all of my endeavors, challenges, and accomplishments. From fishing trips to baseball games, bicycle repairs to bandages, paper airplanes to piano lessons, birthday parties to graduations, my mom and dad are the greatest. I can't even fathom what it would be like for a parent to watch their only child go through such an intense experience. The strength and courage of them was beyond admirable.

THIRD TIME'S A CHARM - MONDAY, JULY 19, 1999

THE PATIENT WAS POSITIONED INTO THE LATERAL POSITION WITH HIS HEAD HELD INTO PLACE BY A FACE AND HEAD HOLDER TO GAIN EASY ACCESS TO THE BULK OF THE PATIENT'S TUMOR. THE AREA OF THE PATIENT'S LEFT PRE-OPERATED SKULL WAS LOCALIZED USING THE BRAIN LAB NAVIGATIONAL SYSTEM. THE AREA WAS SHAVED AND PREPPED IN THE USUAL FASHION.

THE PROPOSED INCISION SITE WAS MARKED WITH A SURGICAL MARKING PEN AT THE PATIENT'S PREVIOUS CRANIOTOMY INCISION SITE AND INFILTRATED WITH LIDOCAINE.

USING A BLADE SCALPEL, A HORSESHOE-SHAPED SKIN INCISION WAS MADE IN THE PREVIOUS INCISION SITE. CLIPS WERE APPLIED TO THE SKIN EDGES TO PROMOTE HEMOSTASIS.

BECAUSE THE PATIENT DID NOT HAVE AN UNDERLYING
BONE FLAP, THE SCALP WAS VERY ADHERENT TO THE
UNDERLYING DURA. THE SCALP WAS CAREFULLY DISSECTED
OFF THE UNDERLYING DURA. THE SKIN FLAP WAS REFLECTED
INFERIORLY AND RAPPED WITH A MOIST LAP PAD THEN
RETRACTED BACK WITH FISHHOOKS AND ELASTIC BANDS.

NEXT, USING SMALL DURAL SCISSORS THE DURA WAS
OPENED IN A U-SHAPED FASHION. PORTIONS OF THE DURA
WERE NOTED TO BE INFILTRATED BY BRAIN TUMOR. UPON
ELEVATION OF THE DURAL FLAP IT WAS NOTED TO BE VERY
INFLAMMATORY AND INFILTRATED BY TUMOR SO THE DURAL
FLAP WAS EXCISED AND SENT TO PATHOLOGY.

AT THIS POINT, THE PATIENT'S TUMOR WAS EASILY
LOCALIZED ON THE SURFACE OF THE BRAIN. BEFORE
RESECTING ANY TISSUE, MOTOR STRIP MAPPING WAS
PERFORMED TO ADEQUATELY LOCALIZE THE MOTOR CORTEX.
AN ELECTRODE GRID WAS PLACED ON THE SURFACE OF THE
BRAIN AND SLID FORWARD UNDER THE DURA TOWARDS THE
PRESUMED MOTOR CORTEX OF THE TUMOR. FROM THERE IT
WAS FELT THAT THE EXTENT OF THE DISSECTION COULD BE
CARRIED OUT SAFELY WITHOUT INJURY TO PRIMARY MOTOR
CORTEX.

THE INTRAOPERATIVE MICROSCOPE WAS THEN
BROUGHT IN TO THE FIELD. USING FORCEPS AND CURVED
MICROSCISSORS, AN INCISION WAS MADE AROUND THE
PERIPHERY OF THE BULK OF THE TUMOR . . .

A little incision here, another resection there. So, this horse walks into a
bar, and the bartender says, "Gee, why the long face?"

. . . FURTHER TUMOR TISSUE AT THE DEPTH OF THE

RESIDUAL CAVITY WERE CAREFULLY EXAMINED USING THE INTRAPOSTOPERATIVE MICROSCOPE. GROSS TUMOR THAT WAS NOTED TO BE SOFT, GRAYISH-YELLOW WAS BIOPSIED AND SENT TO PATHOLOGY FOR FROZEN SECTION. FROZEN SECTION REVEALED CNS LYMPHOMA. AT THIS POINT, THIS AREA OF TUMOR TISSUE WAS RESECTED USING THE SELECTOR ULTRASONIC SURGICAL ASPIRATOR. BLEEDING VESSELS WERE EASILY COAGULATED WITH BIPOLAR FORCEPS. ADDITIONAL TUMOR TISSUE WAS RESECTED ALONG THE LINING OF THE TUMOR CAVITY UNTIL ALL TISSUE THAT WAS GROSSLY ABNORMAL BY VIRTUE OF ITS COLOR, CONSISTENCY OR TEXTURE WAS REMOVED. AT THE DEPTH OF THE TUMOR RESECTION ANTERIORLY, IT WAS FELT THAT THE TOP PORTION OF THE TUMOR CAVITY WAS GETTING RELATIVELY CLOSE TO THE SPEECH SENSORY AREA. BECAUSE OF THIS, THE RESECTION WAS STOPPED BEFORE ENTERING AREAS OF THE ELOQUENT BRAIN.

Dr. Liau was successful in her endeavor, as she resected the optimal amount of remaining tumor without affecting any motor senses. She did a phenomenal job. Going into my brain to get it all may have been absolutely devastating. Her consensus agreed with my first neurosurgeon, Dr. Davis, back in Reno. I may not be able to speak as you read this.

THE RESECTION CAVITY WAS THEN IRRIGATED UNTIL THE RETURN OF IRRIGATING FLUID WAS CRYSTAL CLEAR. OBVIOUS REMAINING BLEEDING POINTS WERE COAGULATED WITH BIPOLAR FORCEPS. THE TUMOR CAVITY WAS THEN LINED WITH SURGICEL TO MAINTAIN HEMOSTASIS AND THE SURGICEL WAS THEN IRRIGATED OUT ONCE NO FURTHER BLEEDING WAS OBSERVED.

THE DURA WAS THEN CLOSED IN A WATER TIGHT FASHION USING SEVERAL SUTURES. BEFORE THE LAST SEVERAL STITCHES WERE PLACED, THE RESECTION CAVITY WAS FILLED WITH SALINE TO PREVENT AIR FROM REMAINING IN THE HEAD. THE BUR HOLE SITES WERE COVERED WITH SMALL PIECES OF GELFOAM TO PROMOTE HEMOSTASIS AND TO PREVENT LEAKAGE OF CSF.

AT THIS POINT, THE CRANIOPLASTY WAS PERFORMED TO REPAIR THE PATIENT'S SKULL DEFECT. A TITANIUM MESH WAS PLACED IN THE CRANIAL DEFECT AND SECURED INTO PLACE WITH SEVERAL TITANIUM SCREWS. CRANIOPLASTY MATERIAL WAS THEN APPLIED INTO THE SKULL DEFECT AND MOLDED TO THE SHAPE OF THE CONTOUR OF THE PATIENT'S SKULL. THIS CRANIOPLASTY MATERIAL WAS ALLOWED TO DRY FOR 20 MINUTES.

AFTER THE PATIENT'S CRANIOPLASTY HAD SET, THE WOUND WAS THEN CLOSED IN MULTIPLE LAYERS. THE TITANIUM CRANIAL FIXTURE WAS SECURED WITH SEVERAL INTERRUPTED SUTURES. THE OVERLYING SKIN WAS CLOSED WITH A RUNNING INTERLOCKING NYLON STITCH. THE WOUND WAS THEN COVERED WITH OINTMENT, TEFLA, AND STERILE GAUZE PADS. A FULL STERILE HEAD DRESSING WAS THEN APPLIED OVER THE PATIENT'S HEAD. THE PATIENT TOLERATED THE PROCEDURE WELL AND THERE WERE NO INTRAOPERATIVE COMPLICATIONS.

When I woke up in the IC unit, I was at peace with myself; not restless or heavily breathing like my first craniotomy at St. Mary's. I was relieved to come out of surgery feeling more like myself. I could even speak more clearly. A major milestone had been reached, as I began to take the upper hand in this battle.

I spent only one day in the intensive care unit to recover from the operation. That was certainly good news, but even better news was the nurse who took care of me. She was hot. The hottest I'd seen since I became ill back in May. I don't remember her name, but she was 29, brunette, single, very attractive, and she babied and adored me. Intensive care had its advantages.

A LONG DAY AND AN EVENING IN HELL - JULY 22

I felt good, and I wanted to go home. The doctors arranged a couple more tests and scans prior to my supposed release. My impression was that I'd be out of the hospital within the next few hours. In the meantime Dad and I walked around outside for some fresh air to escape the infernal hospital, and we entertained ourselves by making stupid jokes. It felt good to vent and inhale fresh air.

There were cement fixtures that served as places to sit. They also served as receptacles to plant trees and other vegetation, which decorated the vicinity of the hospital. Dad and I had already begun to make sarcastic remarks about the hospital. One of the nurses gave me some suppositories just in case I was having trouble defecating. I didn't know what they were used for, but apparently you stick them up your butt to loosen up your digestive tract so you can relieve yourself. I asked my dad what they were supposed to do, and he said, "They loosen up your bowels so you can take a dump."

Then I asked him if he ever had to take one. He said, "Yeah."

I asked, "How was that?"

He replied, "It was a blast."

I burst into uncontrollable laughter and had to walk away in tears to relieve the pressure in my head. We both laughed hysterically.

The day dragged on while I waited for my final calls for a few more tests. I grew restless in my boredom and became easily irritated. There was nothing constructive for me to do. I just wanted to go home, and the longer I stayed in the hospital, the more demoralized I became. Needless to say this was becoming a very long day. At 6:00 p.m. I was finally called for a chest

X-ray. At 7:00 p.m. I was called in for a spinal MRI. By then it was too late to send me home. I would have to stay another night, which was the absolute last thing I wanted to do.

When I received my first couple of MRI's, I couldn't stand them because they were awfully loud and annoying. I was not yet introduced to earplugs. It's a good thing that I was not claustrophobic because those MRI tubes don't allow much room to move around. They are about three feet in diameter and cylindrical. I was just getting used to them when I had to undergo my first spinal MRI.

My previous brain MRIs would last between a half hour to forty-five minutes, and by now I could tolerate them. To my surprise the spinal MRI confined me for two hours, which was absolutely ridiculous. Perhaps if I was notified that the MRI would last two hours, I might not have been so upset about it. I only had a two-minute break within those two hours, not to mention the fact that I just had brain surgery two days earlier. The radiologists didn't even tell me how long it would take, but by the time it was over, I was dead asleep. Then they woke me up again. I was back in my room around 9:15 p.m., very irritated and aware that I would have a final procedure before the day was over.

When I got back to my room after the spinal MRI, it seemed the doctors ascertained that I should have a spinal tap (a.k.a. lumbar puncture) at 10 p.m. I thought spinal tap was the name of a rock band. Well, yeah, but this was no rockin' matter. I noticed a plastic, sealed box with various metal sounds rattling in it as I picked it up to shake around. On the box were pictures of needles about four inches long. That was all I needed to convince myself that the worst may be yet to come. I had a feeling that the term *spinal tap* was going to take on a whole new meaning.

I watched ESPN's *SportsCenter* and browsed through other channels as time passed. It was 11 p.m., and no doctors. I was exhausted. I knew I could go into a vicious deep sleep if I so desired, although I knew that the second I got settled in, I'd be called in for the spinal tap. That's just the way things seemed to work in my time of chaos. Then again, I wasn't adapted to the repetitive spontaneous-stagnant pattern of the hospital merry-go-round. I was so drained I don't think I could have even vented my frustrations into four-letter words. I passed out shortly after 11 p.m.

At approximately 11:45 the door opened. In came a nurse and three doctors. "OK, Daniel, were here to give you a lumbar puncture."

I thought, "Oh. First of all, you're two hours late. Second, why are there four of you? And third, what the hell are you going to do to me?" I was feeling a little crazy, like Jack Nicholson, in *The Shining*, but it would be them who may have been thinking, "We're not going to hurt you, we're just going to bash your brains in."

"Well, what exactly is a lumbar puncture?" I timidly asked.

I don't remember word-for-word what they said, but I was given a summary and sequence of events that would transpire during the actual procedure. I was instructed to curl into a fetal position as tight as possible while laying on my side.

"Like this?" I demonstrated.

"Tighter than that. As tight as you can," someone replied. This would allow a greater opening for the doctor to penetrate a four-inch-long needle into the center of the lower part of my back to draw cerebral spinal fluid (CSF).

They numbed my back with a piercing of lidocaine before initiating the procedure. Within a few minutes the numb effect kicked in. The medical team began making their moves as they instructed me to roll on my side, and squeeze into the tightest ball I thought I could make. Before my back was draped and prepped in the usual sterile manner, the doctor palpated and applied pressure in search for the proper gap in my spinal column. The only nurse who occupied the room offered her hands for me to hold as the procedure transpired. I trembled and squeezed her fingers as the doctor inserted the syringe. So far no pain, but a lot of pressure. I could hear popping noises as the needle began to break into the deeper layers of my spinal column.

Then, like a blind slap in the face, I experienced the worst burst of pain in my life. Apparently there are a lot of nerves in that area. The resident stabbed one while doing the deed. The *son of a bitch* went in crooked.

It was the worst physical pain that I can barely fathom to describe. It was like a surge of electricity that only lasted a second but concentrated through my whole body as if every ounce of pain was a sting from a thousand killer bees. The lumbar needle was then withdrawn and a bandage was placed on the sampled area. The CSF was sent off for culture tests, cell count, glucose, and protein studies.

The worst part about the whole thing was that the doctor who performed the lumbar puncture wasn't yet a doctor. I now know he was a medical student who was getting his experience. No wonder it took three people to supervise him as he prepped and performed the procedure. The physician in training was supposed to inform me and then get my consent to carry out the procedure. He very well may have, but I was so discombobulated as a result of the previous events of the day that I probably didn't care what I was asked. I just wanted to get the day over with. Later I learned there is, however, about a 10 percent chance of hitting a nerve. I just wish I had better control of the odds. It turns out that even if you are a patient, you can also be a guinea pig and not even know it.

My mom later told me that they were waiting for her to leave the waiting room and check out of the hospital. That is the reason the procedure took place so late.

CHAPTER 5

"I DON'T THINK WE'RE IN KANSAS ANYMORE"

THE NEXT DAY - JULY 23

Peacefully, after twelve straight hours of sleep, I was awakened in the late hours of the following morning. If circumstances were any different I would have slept until I was ready to leave. Mom and Dad deserved to be home more than anyone. Fatigue sank in with every effort of movement, but despite my tiredness I would rather be on my way. The night prior was a virtual living hell, and any other feeling of existence seemed satisfactory. Anywhere but the hospital was good enough for me. Spinal fluid results, spinal MRI scans, and the chest X-ray all proved to be clean, which confirmed there was no signs of cancer outside of my brain. I was relieved of my patient obligations later that morning.

That night my parents and I stayed at the Munseys for one last time. They were so helpful as we relayed from Reno to UCLA. I wanted to stay and relax for an additional day, but my folks were anxious to go home. So I reluctantly agreed with them, although another day of rest would have been very therapeutic. Mom and Dad were nostalgic, so they agreed we were better off to depart. Who could blame them? I can't imagine anything worse for a parent to experience than to watch their only child go through what I was going through.

THE STRETCH - SATURDAY, JULY 24

The 472-mile drive home from Los Angeles to Reno was long. My parents were emotionally and physically drained from all the drama at UCLA. They had to keep on their toes more than me as we drove home. There were no guarantees the jaunt would go without incident. Seizures, nausea, vertigo, cardiac and respiratory concerns weighed on all of us. As we proceeded to drive, I was in my own world of mundane feelings, relieved that the battle was over. I locked myself into tunnel vision to stay focused on the road because I was afraid of getting carsick if I closed my eyes.

By the third hour Dad needed a break from driving. In fact we all needed a break. There was a restaurant called Pea Soup Andersen's, which appeared to be a popular rest stop, judging by the overflowing parking lot. Across the street was a Del Taco, which sounded appealing to me at the time, but my dad preferred a nice sit-down restaurant. My mom wasn't particular about either.

We waited for nearly ten minutes to be seated at Pea Soup Andersen's when the hostess sat us down with three menus and said "I'll be back in a couple minutes to take your order." Ten minutes went by, followed by another ten minutes. All of the hustle and bustle in the restaurant was beginning to put me into sensory overload, and I became very agitated and overwhelmed. Still, no one to take our order. If it took 20 minutes for someone to take our order, how much longer would it take for them to prepare our food?

After a few more minutes my tolerance ran dry, and I got up to leave the restaurant for Del Taco. While my dad wanted a nice sit-down meal, I just wanted service and something to satisfy the appetite and mood swings from the Decadron steroids. My dad was upset to leave, and my mom just wanted to make sure we ate something for the remaining 300 miles back to Reno. We ate at Del Taco, where the service was immediate and the food was filling.

A VISION

After eleven arduous hours of driving, worry, and hassle, we arrived home at 8 p.m. without any ER medical drama. We were all drained. Mom and Dad brought all my bags into the house, I sorted everything that was mine, threw it on the floor in my room, strolled to the recliner in the living room, sat down, and wondered what I should do with myself. I wasn't quite ready to go to bed, certainly in no condition to read, strumming my guitar was totally out of the question, and staring at the wall depressed me. There was no happy medium, so I resorted to watching television.

Within recent months television had become a wasteland to me, so in mid-June, between craniotomies, I had deserted the idiot box because it was bad therapy. Recreational or physical activity, such as jogging, hiking, mountain biking, or playing a competitive team sport, was what I was accustomed to in my free time; but a hole in my head constricted my safety in doing such things until UCLA. At that time television enhanced all of my frustrations. I resorted to reading instead.

Flipping through the channels made me dizzy, so I settled for *SportsCenter* and set the remote on the arm of the recliner. There were so many channels on basic cable that I couldn't remember what channels were worth watching. In college watching TV was a rare occurrence, and I wasn't used to the variety of 80 different channels. I didn't know what else to do, but I thought television might be a good way to calm my nerves. However every minute drew me into a deeper restlessness, as I felt an episode of sensory overload coming upon me.

Then, strangely, I had a peak experience. I was at a calm with myself, like I was injected with a dose of euphoria and insight. I thought about grabbing a pen to record my thoughts, but I didn't want to lose the edge. The vision was me in the future, dignified, enlightened, and wise. I felt humility and a fierce calm but wondered what else resided in the deeper mystery. This trance persisted just short of ten minutes, but it felt like a lifetime. My thoughts and feelings were deeper and more profound than I could ever remember. I thought I was focused with my current path in life prior to diagnosis, but maybe I was better off headed somewhere else. Perhaps it was a sign of what was to come.

Although I wasn't on any different medications or any mind-enhancing drugs, I just had another wad of my brain scooped out only four days ago. Then again I was feeling ten times better out of UCLA than I felt out of St. Mary's. I wasn't drugged, just feeling better. After I snapped out of my hypnotic state, I was still on the recliner watching *SportsCenter*. It was like being awakened from a blissful dream, only to forget everything the moment you step into the shower. At least I wasn't in a hospital. I found myself in bed by 10 p.m., and I woke up the next morning feeling calm and enlightened.

MOVING TO THE NEXT PHASE

For the first few days of my recovery, I did very little except eat, sleep, practice guitar, play video games on my Sony PlayStation, and read. I was told that, even if a tumor is benign, it is basic standard for patients who have brain surgery to recover within two to three weeks. This gives time for any swelling of the brain to reduce and allows the patient to regain strength. Taking it easy is the theme here. During the previous two months I had been injected and stuck with so many sharp things I couldn't decide if I was being tortured or punished. The IVs were like bloodsucking leeches. They'd stick to me, gnaw, and suck my blood; then they'd go somewhere else, suck some more blood, and leave a nice, little, swollen scar. My arms and hands were puffy. Rest and recovery were certainly needed.

An affirmative diagnosis on my health had not yet been established. My optimism was far greater than my foresight as to what the chances were that I might have cancer. My priority list remained the same. By next summer I would fulfill my life goal of backpacking Europe, followed by a continuation of bachelorhood and a career in engineering. No reconsideration could hold me from getting back on track with my life. I was in a stage of denial, yet I couldn't help but passively ask myself questions such as, "Am I done with all this medical drama? Do I have cancer? If I do, will I undergo chemotherapy or radiation?" Questions I wasn't prepared to answer and possible answers were just too big and overwhelming for me to consider. I did the best I could to keep the situation simple. I certainly wasn't going anywhere.

A week after the third craniotomy, I realized that I felt better after it than I did before it. I wasn't as restless, and my thoughts were more fluent. I learned the tumor was corrupting my cognitive thinking and affecting the way I felt. My sense of self became much clearer after it was removed. The outcome of the final craniotomy was successful, although there was still tumor tissue remaining. I denied the fact that the tumor tissue was malignant, and I told all who asked that the tumor was benign. Out of all honesty, I didn't have a clue what my prognosis was, but I was certain that there was no way I could have cancer.

Just over a week after I returned from UCLA, I began to feel very weak and out of my senses. I also had another headache that I could not shake off, but other than that I was fine. My dad didn't hesitate to respond to my grievance and brought me to St. Mary's once again. Poor guy. After the usual preadmission merry-go-round, I was brought into a room where I was plugged with an IV line. *So far, not so good.* To make a long story short, it was decided that I should have another spinal tap. I told the doctor about my previous spinal tap at UCLA. He responded with a sarcastic chuckle and said, "A resident did it, huh? Well you won't have to worry about that with me." Actually, he sounded a lot more confident as he told me that he had performed more spinal taps than he could count, and I didn't have anything to worry about. "You can never trust those residents," he concluded.

The doc began preparation, the same as was done at UCLA. There was only one assistant whose job was to hand over the proper tools as needed. I was numbed in my lower spinal column by a quick injection of lidocaine. After a short while, as was done in UCLA, I was instructed to roll onto my side and curl up in a tight ball. This time I curled as tight as I could; tighter than I did in UCLA. With his fingers, he applied pressure in my lower back to feel for the proper gap to insert the needle. Without me knowing, the doctor already began to submerge the needle into my lumbar column. I only felt minor pressure, and before I knew it, he was done. No nerve poking, or anything like it; such a relief. My spinal fluid was sent off for testing, and there was no sign of advancement of disease.

Under Dr. Liau's orders, I was advised not to drive for three months because of a seizure risk. With my dad present at the time of the pronouncement, it looked as though I would be caged until the end of those three months. After my first craniotomies in Reno, they gave me a couple of weeks to be back on the road. I was driving in no time, not excessively but at least I could get myself around.

When I was sixteen, I thought that one of the main privileges of driving was personal freedom; and now that privilege as revoked. Not only was I restricted from driving, I also lived on the other side of town, miles away from the majority of my friends. I was grateful when someone would take me to the movies, out to lunch, on a stroll, or just plain hang out to get me out of the house.

THE MOMENT OF TRUTH – AUGUST 16

Days passed at a rapid rate, and the recommended three-week recovery period from UCLA came to a close. I had no choice but to once again come to terms with my reality. On Monday, August 16, a week following a radiation consultation, a different consultation took place with an oncologist in Reno. Oncologists were around me since day one, but I really didn't even know what an oncologist was, let alone what one did. I was pretty much desensitized from most of the technicalities.

The tumor was conclusively diagnosed as primary central nervous system lymphoma (PCNSL). I didn't know if I had cancer or not because I didn't know what PCNSL was. Dr. Conrath, an oncologist in Reno, was briefed on my case. He geared himself up in the most optimal fashion and was prepared to begin my treatment by Thursday, August 19. He mentioned, "The sooner we can begin to fight this, the better your chances of beating it. It is treatable, but we have to go at it aggressively and right away." I was confused.

"So what exactly *is* that?" I asked. "Cancer?"

He paused . . .

"Yes," he sternly replied in a mild tone.

My mind went into a state of vertigo, and my body filled with numbness. A fear I did not know could be possible was now my reality, and within a moment I was once again in the center of a living hell. In those scorching moments, I never felt so desolate in my own state of mind and desensitized from hope. The reality of what I had ignored had finally caught up to me, and it overcame me like a tsunami. The walls of my ignorance and denial were no more.

Further described, I was diagnosed with T-cell lymphoma. The term *primary* refers to originating in the brain, hence primary. He said, "Their are basically two types: B-cell and T-cell. You're T-cell. Most people who are diagnosed with PCNSL are B-cell. B-cell is very common but T-cell is very rare."

Great. Just great. First I'm diagnosed with a brain tumor the day after I graduate from college. Then I have back-to-back craniotomies, where a hearty portion of my brain was placed in a petri dish to see how the cultures would grow. Third, I get this metal plate implanted in my head to replace a missing chunk of my skull. Next, I am officially diagnosed with a tongue-twister disease, primary central nervous system lymphoma. Then I find out it's cancer. And then it's specifically T-cell lymphoma, the rare form of the disease. I actually felt special because I was a one-of-a-kind–type deal. Until these burning moments, I had never been personally involved or associated with someone whose life was in jeopardy. Shit just got real!

The clock began to tick, and before I knew it, I found myself in another situation of doubt and frustration. Dr. Conrath handed me a nine-page article that described the basic nature of PCNSL, statistics, and how it could be managed. Possible long-term and short-term outlooks were not guaranteed but were meant to prolong a natural life as much as possible. Some statistics were good, some were not so good. Chemotherapy has been recognized as treatment for significant prolonged life in some patients with PCNSL. Being a statistic of "some" isn't very promising.

The conclusion of the article stated the following: "The addition of multidrug chemotherapy to whole-brain radiation appears to prolong survival for patients younger than 60, but the median survival reaches a plateau at approximately 40 months." If I were in the median, I'd be dead before I was even thirty years old. It continued, "Without a commitment to study these regimens formally, the treatment of PCNSL will continue to depend on anecdotal experience, and the median survival is likely to remain disappointingly short."

According to the protocol that Dr. Conrath planned to put me on, I would be poisoned, nuked, and radiated for four months. A grueling ten-week course of chemotherapy appeared like it would consume any discretionary strength in my body. That would be two to three days in the hospital every other week for ten weeks. Immediately following the tenth week of chemo, I would undergo a five-week course of radiation. Each radiation session was set to be five to ten minutes per day, five days a week. At least that would give me a little room to begin gathering myself, but then again my brain would be frying. After that, one more week of treatment would be required before starting remission.

Along with the chemotherapy, I would have what was called an Ommaya reservoir surgically implanted into my head. There, it would be used for easy access into my brain for the admission of chemo drugs. That's bad enough, but even worse, it would be in my head for the rest of my life, however long that would be. Who knows, maybe I could pretend it would be used as a tracking device for the FBI or as a transmitter to the alien mother ship. That would be neat, too. For every impure thought, I would be shocked. If that was the case, I would be dead in no time at all. I couldn't believe what I was bound for within the next months, and the whole idea was making me sick. I was up shit creek without a paddle. One hell of a college graduation gift.

I was advised to seek a second opinion. I had no idea of the various chemotherapy treatments for my disease, nor did I have much time to do substantial research to find the best treatment out there. My parents and I were already exhausted from prior events. Where was I to start looking for the answers to questions I didn't know to ask? I only had two days to decide. Mom, Dad, and I were at the same level, which was frightened and lost. Who the hell knows what to do when all of a sudden, someone says, "You have cancer."?

I had very little knowledge of the effects of chemotherapy. The only thing I thought I knew about it was that I would probably lose my hair, become extremely skinny, and hate everything. Chemotherapy involves toxic drugs that are flushed through the body to kill, slow down, or stop the growth of cancer cells. It can be a grueling and weary process but essential to get through for prolonged wellness. That was the first thing I learned about chemotherapy. I wasn't looking forward to the inevitable anguish I would have to suffer for four months, but I would have to take the bull by the horns for a fighting chance. My effort and motivation to seek alternatives and second opinions was beginning to dwindle, due to exhaustion and frustration.

Another concern was the undefined statistics regarding radiation and its long-term effects on the brain. Would I still be able function as a cognitive person in five years? To be honest, I wasn't convinced Dr. Conrath's treatment, coupled with my lack of knowledge, would ensure me with the confidence to maintain long-term vision and certainty in my life. There had to be something more promising than this.

Time was running out, and action had to take place. Dr. Conrath seemed to be a pretty good guy from what I knew of him, but a day is hardly a respectable amount of time to get to know someone. Conrath admitted, "I know that I don't know much about you, nor do you know much about me. I advise you to venture for a second opinion because I know this is something you'd like to put behind you, but at the same time you can't put it off. I'm surprised it took this long to start chemotherapy," he said.

Dr. Conrath sounded a little aggravated that it took three weeks before the doctors in UCLA got me going with chemotherapy. He thought I should have been on chemo a week earlier. I respected Dr. Conrath for being up-front with me. "The sooner we can start treating you, the better your chances of success."

I decided to save myself the grief of indecision and committed my faith to Dr. Conrath. I slept very little that night. The following morning I woke up feeling very discouraged and empty. Later that day I was contacted by an oncologist from the medical team that dealt with me in UCLA. His name was Dr. Cloughsey, and he was evidently up-to-date on my case. There were so many doctors walking around UCLA, and I had such a short-term memory that, even if I did meet him, I wouldn't recognize him. My dad testifies I met him, but I don't have the slightest memory of it. Nonetheless, I was impressed with the end result from Dr. Liau, and I was all ears to hear what Dr. Cloughsey had to say.

THE PACKAGE

A couple of weeks after my return home from UCLA, I received a package in the mail that was the size of a shoebox. It was from my cousin Christine Munsey. Inside the *Van's* shoebox were several random, yet comforting, items, including seashells, a butterfly ornament, a picture frame, a book called *Jonathan Livingston Seagull*, a couple of candles, a piece of surf wax, and a letter.

I didn't have siblings, but Christine was my only relative who was closest to my age. The letter touched my heart as she described the contents in the box:

> *I had a few hours of quality time in my house, so I decided to get out my craft supplies and get creative. I wanted to get you something, but what? I remembered in high school when I was going through a rough time with my parents, family, school, you name it, my brother slipped me a dirty old piece of wax that smelled like Coca-Cola. He told me it was his good luck charm that helped him through tough times. For*

many years after, when times were shitty, somehow, someway, picking up this dirty piece of wax and smelling it was very comforting. Now it's time to pass it on. I know it won't cure you, but maybe when you pick it up you will know that I think about you often.

The book is a short story; it's one of my favorite books. Read it and enjoy it. I really regret not being able to spend more time with you while you were visiting. I have so much to talk to you about. You're the only one in my family that is remotely close to my age, which is fun for me. Anyways, remember I'm thinking of you. Get well. Now!!!

Luv Always,
Your Cuz Christine

The scent of the Coca-Cola surf wax was a healing elixir in itself. *Jonathan Livingston Seagull* was a short read but was one of the most inspirational books I've ever read. It's about a seagull who had a dream of flying faster than any other seagull, and no matter how many times he crashed in the ocean, he never gave up. No other seagull in the flock believed in him, and he was ostracized and ridiculed. But when he learned to control his flight, he became the leader of the flock.

CHAPTER 6

FIRST IS THE WORST

Lance Armstrong would go on to win his first Tour de France in July of 1999. Aunt Melva mailed the newspaper clipping to me and it gave me a great sense of hope.

DOMINO EFFECT – AUGUST 17, 1999

Tuesday morning, August 17, the day after I was informed of my potential death sentence, Dr. Cloughsey from UCLA called my house. He had a very cool, confident voice when he told me, "There is a treatment in Portland, Oregon, called the Blood Brain Barrier Disruption. It's chemotherapy that doesn't involve radiation." As Celebrity Chef *Emeril* would say, "*BAM.*" I was sold, plain and simple.

Dr. Cloughsey and I spoke briefly before I handed the phone to my dad. He was filled in with more comprehensive details. Relief consumed my mind. When the conversation ended, I said, "I'm doing that, and that's all there is to it."

"OK, OK. Just hold your horses," he responded. By now I had the utmost respect for the advancement of medicine at UCLA.

Based on positive outcomes within recent years, Dr. Cloughsey became convinced that the Blood Brain Barrier Disruption (BBBD) is a reasonable, alternative form of treatment. He believed that, when it came to dealing with PCNSL, especially for young patients like myself, I'd stand a better chance for a better quality of life and longer survival. My young and strong body could withstand high doses of chemotherapy. It wasn't that I wanted chemotherapy, but it was a better outlet than radiation. Apparently Dr. Cloughsey had been following the BBBD program closely, and I would be the first patient ever referred from UCLA to Oregon Health Science University's (OHSU) BBBD program. Dad became my relay man to share this information with family.

Beginning with Dr. Conrath, the next four days were a chain reaction of vital events. Monday was when I first met Dr. Conrath and learned I had cancer, the most frightening moment of my life. That night I weighed the options, and I succumbed to his treatment. I was cornered, and it seemed there was no way out. The next day Dr. Cloughesy called with news to ease my soul. Tuesday night, plane reservations were made. On Wednesday evening my dad and I flew to Portland. Because the flight was booked on such short notice, we had to pay a hefty sum for airplane tickets. Thursday was when my dad and I would gather more understanding of the BBBD Program.

AUGUST 18

I have little recollection of many specifics during that first visit. My brain and short-term memory were nowhere near recovered from the craniotomies, and it was very difficult to absorb details. Much of my recollection was outlined in a OHSU/BBBD consent form and a patient information video.

The BBBD program was pioneered in 1982, actively practiced, and directed by a very dedicated man, Dr. Edward Neuwelt in Portland, Oregon. It is a treatment that only involves chemotherapy in hopes that radiation won't have to be an option in the long haul; that was enough information to convince me that OHSU is the place to be. Knowing that I could kill the cancer cells in my brain without radiation to preserve my cognitive mind was exciting indeed. I willingly and confidently accepted the alternative.

The program is intended to prolong a patient's survival and also to improve the quality of life during treatment. In the call of duty, the program takes a comprehensive approach for patients and their families, which includes dealing with complex emotional, personal, and psychological needs.

Prior to my being referred to the BBBD program, I was treading deep water. If I didn't swim in one direction soon, I would most likely drown in a sea of uncertainty. The second opinion Dr. Conrath suggested I seek was inadvertently delivered to me on a silver platter and not a day too soon. The BBBD patrol rescued me, brought me to higher ground, and instantly gave me the confidence and foresight to continue my journey through life. Instead of the original aggressive approach suggested by Dr. Conrath, the Blood Brain Barrier Disruption seemed to be a more forgiving form of treatment and deemed to be superior in its prolonged effectiveness. The duration of chemotherapy would stretch over the course of an entire year, but the time given to regather and advance after each treatment would offset being overwhelmed and disoriented.

On a month-to-month basis, the BBBD typically requires a four-day stay in the hospital. Day one is for preadmission, physical examination, MRI or CT scan to mark the status of my tumor, a chest X-ray, an EKG, and other preliminary tests that may be required. Other tests included hearing, sight, and neurological examinations. On days two and three, the BBBD is performed, with a twenty-four-hour gap between each disruption. Expected to be feeling good, day four is the day of release from OHSU and my return flight back to Reno.

A long list of complications from the treatment's earlier years were listed on a consent form. Among them were blood clots, injured arteries, high blood pressure, infections due to low white blood cell counts, high-frequency hearing loss, and brain stem injury. One patient died because of excessive intracranial pressure. Obviously, reading the disclaimer was nerve racking, but it seemed to be the best thing around. I hoped to come out with minimal or no mental or physical deficits. My only sense of control was my attitude and a passiveness to the medical reality. There was absolutely no point in me obsessing, unless I wanted to be completely miserable.

Mountain Biking - Summer 1995

When I was a junior in high school, my GT Timberline mountain bike was sto-
len from my garage. My dad would go to work early in the morning but seldom closed the garage door. Just over an hour after he left for work, I would
be off to school, and I closed the automatic door on my way out. In the
garage my bike was the only thing of value to me. I kept it locked to a bench
post. It just so happened that the night before the theft, I tuned up my GT
so I could ride it the following afternoon. I forgot to lock it up that night and
didn't realize it was gone until I returned from school the next day. After
realizing something was missing, I became irate, felt violated, and reported
the theft to the police. There was no further trace beyond the tire tracks that
streaked across our front lawn.

Until my first summer of college, I hadn't ridden because I couldn't
afford to buy a new bike. By this time I was a resident of the Pi Kappa Alpha
fraternity house and was initiated as an active member the semester before.
One of my fraternity brothers, Lorin Darst, owned a Diamond Back mountain bike. The bike sat in the basement, unmoved and dusty, for as long as
I could remember. We exchanged favors. I repaired the bike's two flat tires,
greased the gears, and realigned the brake pads. Lorin appreciated the
favor and didn't mind me riding it. I was anxious to ride, as it was the beginning of summer.

With every passing week, I explored new trails at all corners of town
and found myself riding deeper into the hills on each ride. Two of the advantages of living in Reno are the short drive to Lake Tahoe and the abundant,
easily accessible jeep trails and single-track trails for riding. At the time, one
of my favorite treks was an approximate 15-mile round trip to 3,000-year-
old petroglyphs known as the Pah Rah petroglyphs. There, I have seen
small herds of wild antelope, horses, various desert reptiles, cattle, and the
strangest looking bugs I've ever seen. Midsummer thunderstorms are like
angry Indian spirits pounding their drums. When clouds subside and the

smell of fresh rain lingers, brilliant sunsets engulf the open solitude. Colors of orange, red, pink, and yellow form random patterns of infinite variety.

My most common ride, however, was a generous mix of single-track and jeep trails known as Keystone Canyon. Keystone Canyon begins with almost one mile of wash then switches to single-track. For the next four miles, jeep trails and single-track cross each other. I'd make an effort to explore different roads and trails on every ride. On average, I'd ride 15-20 miles twice a week. At the time I held down a full-time job during the summer, and mountain biking was a great way for me to unwind.

In general riding a bike during a thunderstorm, especially in an open desert, isn't the wisest of choices for recreational activities. As common sense dictates, where there is thunder, there is lightning. One afternoon during the hot month of August, thunderheads were merging over the horizon. It's the time of year when temperatures linger in the mid-nineties to low hundreds, and strings of thunderstorms aren't uncommon. They are appreciated as much as they are feared because of lightning strikes that can lead to forest fires and brush fires.

As I rode on this particular day through Keystone Canyon, rain began to trickle when I reached the seven-mile mark. Thunder became louder and lightning streakier. Clouds within my peripheral vision became darker, yet I persisted. I was at the point of no return, and if I turned back, I would be rained on no matter what. The atmosphere was galvanized, and here I was, alone in the great wide open on an aluminum-framed bike. *I was the perfect conductor.* Almost instantly I was pelted by massive, marble-sized raindrops as I reached the peak of a respectable-sized, contoured knoll. The route I took was off of my usual beaten path. Within minutes I was soaked to the bone, my wet T-shirt leeched to my skin like spandex. I peeled it off and stuffed it to dangle out of my shorts. There was nowhere for me to run or hide. I was in an extreme state of living, and I was loving every moment of it.

The combination of elation, adrenaline, and a sense of fear gave me chills and motivated me to pedal faster and harder. Gnarly bolts of lightning painted the sky as far as the eye could see. Crackling thunder smashed my ears, as every hair on my body made a valiant attempt to stand up under the goose bumps that tingled along my drenched body. For several minutes I rode high on adrenaline, but despite the rush, the bulk of the storm passed me as fast as it came. I continued to ride until the high tapered off. Eventually I made it home.

ADMIT ONE

MONTH I: AUGUST 29 – SEPTEMBER 26

When my dad and I flew up to Portland on Sunday evening, we were fortunate to have a free place to stay. The American Cancer Society (ACS) hooked us up with a room at a Marriott hotel in downtown Portland. Airfare, on the other hand, was something we couldn't avoid. Along with my mom, who would arrive the following evening, we would fly from Reno to Portland and back once a month for my chemo.

Dad studied the TriMet transit system days prior to our departure from Reno. TriMet is comprised of subway and bus lines. Our hotel was downtown, where the heart of the transit system resides. The only thing we had to do was walk to the bus stop and the number-8 bus would take us to OHSU. The buses ran every 15 minutes on the weekdays, so we didn't have to worry too much about being late.

I slept poorly that Sunday night, and waking up the following Monday morning was difficult. I was not acclimated to the Pacific Northwest climate, which seemed to leave me sluggish. My dad and I knew we'd be late because I tend to sleep in, especially if I'm tossing and turning the night before. Since we were already late, I requested that we grab a decent breakfast at the hotel restaurant downstairs. I had a freshly made omelet, while Dad had the same, along with French toast. Due to my own indolent pace, we were nearly an hour late.

Preadmission, necessary tests, and procedures took place as the day began. A nurse by the name of Janeele introduced herself with a friendly smile and proceeded to ask a series of questions regarding complications, comments, and other medical history. She soon stuck me in the forearm with an IV that would remain until I was released. It was my central line for chemo and blood draws. As the day dragged on, I tried to sleep as much as possible to burn a few unnecessary hours. My dad and I ate dinner at the hospital before Mom's plane arrived in Portland later that evening. She had to work that day.

Shortly after I returned to my hospital room, a nurse instructed me to shave my pelvic area. One of the human body's main arteries is located in that area, and it's called the femoral artery. During treatment a catheter would be inserted into the femoral artery and would eventually go to the back of my brain. Not much else went on that night. I was hooked to an IV bag and monitor at 9 p.m. to maintain an adequate level of fluid. The nurse came in at random intervals to check in and to feed me a colorful concoction of pills, including the antiseizure medication, Dilantin. The look of them alone made me sick, so I downed them with one cup of water and forgot about it. I was told that I would be the first of four patients to be treated early the next morning.

Mom and Dad left the hospital shortly before 10 p.m. so they could catch the last evening bus back to the hotel. They were certain to be back in the morning for my first round of chemotherapy. Meanwhile I briefly talked to the patient across from me, but I don't remember what we talked about. I watched TV on a little TV: from the wall perpendicular to my pillow was a retractable arm with a tiny, five-inch-screen television at the end.

I wasn't allowed to eat or drink after midnight. It was all good because, once the foreign chemicals fused through my body, I lost my appetite. Uncomfortable is the word that best defines trying to sleep in a hospital. My memory of detail is vague during those nights because I was medicated and hooked to an IV. To enhance the discomfort, a mild aura of hospital odor, footsteps back, forth, up, and down the hall and people coughing in other rooms added to the foreign environment. An occasional *beep* from my IV pole when my IV bag ran low didn't help much. All I wanted to do was fall asleep so I could avoid thinking about the stale surroundings.

The following morning, just before seven, I awakened feeling slightly sedated. I had to take a big leak, but my balance was shaky. Mom and Dad were there, like they said they would be. I required assistance from my mom and the nurse to escort me to the restroom while dragging my IV pole through the obstacle course of a bed, chair, and the door. I was cautious about tugging the IV in my arm. During my moment of privacy, I stripped off the remainder of my clothes in exchange for a hospital gown. The nurse and my mom were outside the door, waiting to assist me out of the restroom and back onto the bed.

A small cup of water and more pills were waiting when I returned to sit on the edge of my bed. My body was so infiltrated with sedatives and my mouth dehydrated of all pleasant sensory feeling that the water tasted bland. I felt slightly nauseous but not quite to the brink where I would vomit—although with a little physical exertion, I'm convinced that I could have done it.

I was informed that an escort would soon arrive with a gurney to haul me into the chemo room. All BBBD patients were placed in ward 5A, which is where I would sleep every night while at OHSU. When it was my time for treatment, transport wheeled me to the tenth floor of the same building, the South Hospital. My parents were with me each step of the way. From there I was rolled down a hall to a mystery door, where chemotherapy would take place within. My family and I said our brief good-byes along with hugs before I was slowly rolled into the angiography suite. Angiography is an X-ray survey of the internal anatomy of the body and blood vessels.

Much like my initial feelings of my first craniotomy, I felt strange and out of place as I was rolled into the room. I didn't recognize anyone. From my gurney I was assisted to slide over to the operating table, feeling like an abductee from *The X-Files*. Although I had already survived three craniotomies, I was still uncomfortable about being put to sleep. Instead of cutting into my head, I was about to be poisoned by chemotherapy rat poison. The anesthesiologist introduced himself and told me what the procedure would entail. A breathing mask was lightly placed over my nose and mouth. After a few seconds the mask was pressed snuggly onto my face so the only thing I could inhale was the gas. Slowly my eyes began to flutter as I tried my hardest not to fall asleep. I managed to resist for about 20 seconds, but once I was out . . . I was out.

The Low-Down

Since 1982 Dr. Neuwelt and the BBBD program have been extensively researching the effective delivery of chemotherapy drugs for treating various brain cancers. BBBD is chemotherapy received both intravenously and intra-arterially, and it requires general anesthesia. While asleep, the doctors begin to do the work. A four-inch needle adjacent to a catheter is threaded into the femoral artery in the pelvis area just above the hip. When the needle is filtered into the artery, it is removed, leaving the catheter in place. Under angiography, the catheter is slowly guided through the body, passed around but not into the heart, and finally into the neck arteries, where chemotherapy bombards the tumor. After 24 hours the same thing is done through the other side of the groin area to either the other side or the back portion of the brain.

During this short but intense process, critical procedures are accomplished to ensure optimum outcome. When the catheter reaches the brain, a concentrated sugar solution, mannitol, is infused to open the tight junctions of the blood-brain barrier. The blood-brain barrier is the brain's natural defense, composed of tightly knitted cells that line the walls of the blood vessels in the brain. The tightly knit cells create a barrier that blocks the entry of various substances, including many therapeutic agents. By temporarily shrinking these cells with mannitol, the barrier may be opened, allowing chemotherapy drugs to pass into the brain and reach the tumor. Compared with standard chemotherapy, BBBD therapy increases the delivery of the chemotherapy drugs to the tumor and to the surrounding area of the tumor by tenfold to one-hundred fold.

The first BBBD for any new patient is a learning experience for everyone. No one knew how I'd respond during or after my first treatment. Obviously I felt nothing during the procedure because I was asleep. Wednesday did not exist. I woke up Thursday midmorning, thinking that it was still Tuesday. I felt disoriented, my vision was distorted, and I wasn't quite sure why. Generally the protocol is two disruptions with a 24-hour gap in between, but I was an exception to the rule. Consequently a seizure transpired during the first operation. The doctors needed to monitor my recovery for safety precautions. Intensity and frequency of seizures varies from patient to patient, while some never have seizures during their year of chemotherapy. Hopefully I wasn't among the more-frequent group.

On the final day of my four-day stint at OHSU, a counter-chemotherapy drug called Leucovorin was given to me. It was administered intravenously early in the morning. After the first dose and the passing of six hours, the method typically becomes oral in the form of a pill. Leucovorin is used to prevent the harmful effects of some cancer medicines that are given in high doses. If the chemotherapy isn't stabilized immediately with proper doses of Leucovorin every six hours, the toxicity of the chemotherapy may conform to the body's natural functions, thus creating unwanted complications further down the road. By following direct doctor's orders, 99 to 100 percent of the toxicity of treatment should be out of the body within a week. To Mom and Dad I was fragile as an egg. We were at opposite ends of the spectrum: they were nerve-racked about my safety, while I remained calm yet slightly out of it. I didn't feel too mentally unstable but still a little discombobulated with my vision slightly blurred.

The first evening my parents and I arrived home, we found relief in every aspect except for one tiny thing: a little pill called Leucovorin—forty of them, actually. We had none. I didn't know, but my dad sure did. Evidently we were supposed to pick up a four-day supply at the OHSU pharmacy, but my mom had forgotten in the midst of all the medical drama. There were so many meticulous, new details, in such a foreign environment.

The necessary protocol for Leucovorin is twenty doses, or forty pills. From my end of the spectrum, I had no idea how important it was, but Mom and Dad did. They knew I was two hours late for my dose, and they argued, blaming each other for not having everything together. Finally, Dad called OHSU for the nurse on call. Rose Marie was the on-call nurse who instructed us to drive to the local hospital and order enough to last me through the night and following morning.

Back to St. Mary's we went to pick up the magic medicine. Hopefully they had it. We found our way to the pharmaceutical supply room, where it appeared that the attendant was about to call it a night. After explaining our needs, it took about ten minutes to scrounge a few pills. Apparently their supply was low, but I managed to get enough to last me for another day. With a Dixie cup of water, my dad insisted that I swallow the dose on-site. The pharmaceutical technician said, "You know, each one of those pills is $25." My draw dropped. That multiplies to a month's supply for $1,000. I had to take Leucovorin every six hours, which would make my next dose at 3 a.m. Alarms were set in both my room and my parent's, but they ended up being unnecessary because I tossed and turned all night long. If I dozed off, it was only for a few minutes.

The Decadron didn't help much with my longing for sleep. It was another mandatory supplement prescribed to take every six hours. Things could have been much easier if the time to take the Decadron and Leucovorin wasn't offset by two hours. This meant I could sleep for two hours, wake up, take Decadron, go back to sleep, wake up at three in the morning, take Leucovorin, sleep, wake up two hours later to take Decadron once again, and so on. Decadron was necessary for me because it reduced the swelling of the affected tissue on my brain.

If I was lucky, I may have slept for an hour that night. I woke up the next morning feeling drained and very sleep-deprived. It wasn't even twenty-four hours since I'd been back home. I had it bad, I thought, but I had no idea what else was in store for me.

CHAPTER 7

TRY WALKING IN MY SHOES

TO WIN THE WAR, YOU MUST WIN THE BATTLES

Upon returning home from my first week of BBBD, injecting myself with a drug called Neupogen was required to increase my white blood cell count. I have learned that when the body goes through high doses of chemotherapy, it requires time to rebuild its immune system so that chances of infection are reduced. Chemotherapy kills or paralyzes cancer cells. The bad news is it also affects good cells, a reason why hair falls out on certain patients. It affects the white blood cells that make up the body's immune system, which fights off potential infections and viruses. Chemotherapy also affects red blood cells, which give the body energy. The good news is that both white and red cells can be replenished in time through diligent home care.

The Leucovorin incident on my first return trip home was pretty bad, but grief only escalated the following day. During my first month of chemo, Neupogen brought dreadful adventures to my home medical care. Before administering by way of injection, the drug needs to remain refrigerated. If the Neupogen is foggy, then it is no good. It should be crystal clear. Before I knew what it was, my parents were informed and instructed at OHSU on how this drug should be delivered at home. First prepare a syringe, disinfect the site of injection with an alcohol pad, and pinch a piece of skin on the site. Next, stick the needle into the skin as if throwing a dart, inject the Neupogen, pull out, and provide temporary pressure on the site. For my dad and myself, this was easier said than done. He did not want to stick me with a needle, nor did I want to get stuck.

Dad knew the basic procedure from the instructions he received at OHSU, but I sure as hell wasn't ready to poke myself. I asked my father,

"What's the whole deal with preparing the syringe?"

In a slow, meticulous voice Dad said, "You pull the plunger, about a half inch, like so. Insert the syringe into the vial as dead center as you can. Turn the apparatus upside-down, and push the plunger as far as it will go. Then, by letting go of the plunger, a vacuum effect takes place, causing the Neupogen to transfer into the syringe." Once that was done, he flicked it a couple times to minimize air bubbles. I chose to have the injection on my thigh. Dad wiped an alcohol pad around the target injecting area to disinfect the skin.

The moment had arrived, and I was pretty damn nervous; and to a relative degree he was, too. I could sense my prolonging agony as my thoughts and expressions were very ordinary and repetitive. "OK," I said, "so you're going to pinch a little chunk on my thigh and poke me with the needle?" over and over again. I would have been much more comfortable with a doctor or nurse.

"Yes, that's what I'm going to do," he answered.

Just as he was on the verge of doing the deed, I said "Wait," causing him to stop. I was nervous, and he got annoyed.

"OK, fine . . . if you're not going to let me do it, then I'll let you do it." I timidly responded, "No. No, that's OK."

Finally, he got fed up with my whining and demanded to do it. I looked away as he pinched a piece of skin on my leg and stuck me with the needle. I barely felt the poke, but a slight burn when the Neupogen was injected into my leg. It only last three seconds at the most. Dad gave me a piece of gauze to hold the area down with adequate pressure, as he properly disposed of the syringe. He asked if I wanted to do the second shot, which was Lovenox, a blood thinner that helps prevent blood clots. "It's easy. Just do the same thing I did." Instead of preparing the syringe like Neupogen, the syringe was already prepared.

I said, "Maybe tomorrow."

When tomorrow arrived, I felt relatively confident about stabbing myself with a needle without assistance. I told him to leave the room and I'd do it myself; I needed a minute or two to psyche myself up for the procedure, but after much contemplation, I psyched myself out. I sat there with a three-quarter-inch needle in one hand while pinching a piece of skin in the other. I couldn't bring myself together to poke my own body. This continued for several minutes. I retreated to take a few deep breaths to rebuild my composure, but the moment the tip of the syringe grazed my skin I became nervous and agitated from what seemed to be a simple process. Just stick the stupid thing into my leg and that was it, but it wasn't that simple at the time. My dad went to another room to preoccupy himself while he waited for me to do the deed, and he kept asking me about every ten minutes, "Did you do it?"

"Yeah, just give me a minute," I would say, as if I had it under control.

Almost an hour had passed without progress. Finally my dad came in and demanded to do it himself. I sat there, feeling petrified of stabbing myself with a damn needle. I would sit there for minutes with the tip of the syringe on my skin. The more I thought about it, the more I didn't want to do it. I would retreat back to square one, take a few deep breaths, and rebuild composure again and again and again.

The senseless fear was something I couldn't control no matter how hard I tried, but I guess there was something about making holes in my body that I did not like. For the next three days I played this game, putting myself through the same cycle. Something had to be done soon because I wasn't going to put myself through this anguish for the next twelve months. There had to be another way.

When Monday came around, my dad had to go back to work, and I was on my own for Neupogen and Lovenox shots. Mom was home, but I wasn't about to hand her the responsibility. Instead I resorted to calling Dr. Conrath's office and explaining my dilemma to one of the nurses. She gave me sympathy and told me to come to the office, where I could get some coaching. I arrived shortly thereafter with my mom.

The nurse told me there was an easier way of giving myself injections. I told her about my hesitant attitude and what was happening in my thought process. She was very understanding and explained that a lot of patients have a hard time doing this. She said, "Even after being coached, some patients still can't do it, and someone would always have to do it for them." If I could find any alternative to keeping my dad and me from the grief of poking myself with a needle, I would most willingly accept it.

Nice and slow was the method she taught me, compared to the quick and painless method my dad was performing on me. Quick and painless seemed to be the obvious way to do this, but with nice and slow I know I'd have more control and precision. The nurse instructed me to slowly push the syringe onto the sight of injection until the needle sank in. Still, I was hesitant, but there is something about a woman's nurturing nature that is calming and convincing. Slowly I pressed the syringe into my leg, barely feeling a thing. Then she instructed me to adjust my fingers to where I could push the plunger. Slowly I injected the Neupogen, released the grip of skin, pulled out the needle, and applied moderate pressure to the site until there was no sign of bleeding. That method allowed me to be self-sufficient, and I was able to perform the remaining week's shots on my own.

REVENGE OF THE NEUPOGEN

On the first Wednesday after my first month of chemo, my mom took me to lunch at *On the Border* restaurant around two o'clock that afternoon. We spent a good hour in quality conversation until we decided to depart. My appetite was hearty that day, allowing me to eat a bowl of chips and salsa, two jalapeno-chicken enchiladas, beans, vegetables, and anything else that wasn't liquid. If my plate were to be any cleaner, I would have had to lick it like a dog. As I walked out the restaurant doors to the car, I felt a little lethargic, perhaps because I ate so much Mexican food.

The discomfort departed and consistently came back seemingly every hour. At roughly seven o'clock that evening, the feeling came and went in more frequent intervals, each lapse more intense than the previous one, yet I didn't know what it was or how to react.

I went to my room, rested on my back, and tried reading. About five minutes later I felt a bite on my lower back . . . then again, and again. I got up, left my room, and began pacing around the house. It seemed the longer I sat around, the more the pain increased. I laid on the loveseat for about three seconds until I twitched in pain once again, which instigated me to stand up and pace back and forth. While walking around, I could feel it becoming more intense in intervals between five and ten seconds. My dad was camped on the recliner, watching me do this chicken walk on my tiptoes.

"What's wrong?" he asked. I couldn't muster up words to respond because the episode was so unusual.

"I don't . . . I don't know. My back is just killing me right now." I sat down again, and I was bewildered by this unknown pain. I began writhing in tears and continued to pace to fight it off. Unable to find a solution, Dad went to the phone and called OHSU. In the meantime my mom was conversing on the phone with one of her friends. She seemed to be enjoying her conversation, so I didn't want to bother her because she worried enough about me. My dad called OHSU, and the nurse on call was Rose Marie. I explained what was going on. She answered that it was the Neupogen.

Rose Marie explained, "When you go though chemotherapy, your white blood cell count goes down. Neupogen brings you back up. It takes a couple of days for it to kick in, but once it does, the white blood cells multiply at an exponential rate—so fast that it hurts." The pain pulsated from my lower back, similar to having a spinal tap every ten seconds. The only difference was that it was centralized in my lower back rather than radiating through my entire body.

Rose Marie said I could take some Tylenol to help ease the pain. I popped an extra-strength tablet as soon as I hung up the phone but continued pacing. Ten minutes later the bone pain started to dissipate, and eventually I was able to sit down with a sigh of relief. My mom finished her conversation and came into the living room, where my dad and I were watching TV. She observed the expression on my face, and from her maternal instincts she immediately knew something was wrong. I told her what happened, and she seemed disgruntled that I didn't let her know while the bone pain was happening. By the time the episode ended, I was exhausted. At my next visit to OHSU, two and a half weeks later, I was told that some people are put on morphine because the pain is so unbearable.

Extra strength Tylenol would become another part of my regimen.

BONAFIDE

Two months after my third craniotomy, I was happy to see my hair growing back, full and thick. About three-quarters of an inch overall. It was even starting to cover the inverted horseshoe scar on my head. Things were looking good, but too much optimism would only set me up for disappointment, so I tried to ignore the fact that one day I would have a full head of hair again. Sometimes, when you expect something to happen, it's not as dramatic when it does. I must admit that I was a little shook up when my hair began to fall out because I never imagined what it would be like.

One evening while showering, I noticed gobs of hair accumulating in my hands as I scrubbed my head. My hands looked like they were covered in a thin coat of fur. After I rinsed the hair off my hands, I thought that it may detach itself a little at a time. The next time I went to scrub my head, there was even more hair in my hands. Hair fell from all parts of my body. I've heard of people getting hairy palms from other things, but this was ridiculous. After stepping out of the shower, I began to dab my head dry with a towel. It was a nice, clean towel until I finished the initial scrub, then the towel was covered with thousands of splinters of dead hair. I was speechless. The following morning I woke up and took a look at my blue pillow and noticed another couple thousand pieces of severed hair. After shampooing that night, I knew I was going to be completely bald sooner or later. My head was beginning to look like an ocean with many small islands. "Fuck it," I said bitterly and shaved the rest my head with clippers. I was now a full-blown cancer patient.

The Leash - Sports

Sports have always been an important part of my life. They helped develop my confidence, competitive nature, and team spirit. Since T-ball they also taught me timeless life lessons.

LESSON #1: TRY THE BEST YOU CAN.

I was eight years old when I began playing T-ball as a second baseman. I'll never forget the time I fielded my first ground ball and threw the runner out at first base. Everybody cheered, and I felt like a rock star.

LESSON #2: BE A GOOD SPORT.

We were the Cubs and, win or lose, we'd always shake hands with the opposing team. There weren't too many egos in second grade.

LESSON #3: HAVE FUN.

Even if we lost, there were always postgame snacks and drinks like Twinkies, HoHo's, granola bars, soda, juice boxes, or Capri Sun drinks. Pizza parties were always one of our favorites because we got to go to Round Table Pizza, where we would play arcade games and the jukebox, playing "Jump" by Van Halen over and over again.

The following two years I played in Little League minors as an outfielder and first baseman. The two seasons after that, I played Little League majors at second base, shortstop, and pitcher for the Mariners. My curveball was the best in the league, and I was selected for the Little League all-star team in my district. I also hit my first home run that same year, in sixth grade. It was a line drive over the center field fence. Our all-star team placed third in the county. For the next three seasons, until my sophomore year in high school, I continued to play Babe Ruth at third base, shortstop, and pitcher. In high school I went on to play varsity baseball as a sophomore, junior, at third base and pitcher.

My parents signed me up for league basketball and tennis when I was in elementary school, and I began snow skiing in middle school. In addition to baseball I would be active in all four sports through high school and even played varsity tennis as a senior.

I continued playing sports in college through the Pi Kappa Alpha fraternity. Greek sports were as competitive as any other league sports, especially among rival fraternities. I quickly picked up volleyball, which became my passion sport in league play indoors, on the grass, and at the beach. Seasonal sports such as basketball, softball, tennis, floor hockey, and water polo also consumed my time in extracurricular activities.

My cancer ordeal kept me from participating in any active sporting activities, at least until Dr. Liau patched the hole in my head. Even then, any physical activity would need to be non- or minimal contact. But my chemo leash was about to become even shorter and tighter.

If I wasn't bitten by a slithering IV and numbed by its venomous sedatives, I was leeched with needles that sucked my blood. When I returned home from my first month of chemo, I hoped for a change. Needle scars wrought havoc on my hands, causing swelling and sensitivity. Polka-dot tattoos were results from countless IV hookups and blood draws during times of craniotomies and chemotherapy. IVs would go anywhere there was a vein. While at UCLA I recall once having three IVs connected to my two poor arms. Sometimes a nurse couldn't get the IV to connect with a vein, and I'd be pierced again as a result. Half of the time my hands would get puffy because the IV couldn't infuse or draw. I was afraid to bend my arms for fear that the IV would break in my forearm. It was demoralizing.

To help resolve my dilemma, I was introduced to a chemotherapy accessory called a portacatheter, or central line. During my first hospitalization at OHSU, the device was described to me, and I would need to have one for chemotherapy. A portacatheter is surgically placed under the skin into the subclavian vein, two inches below the collarbone. The location of the port goes into a chosen side of the chest area. I chose the left side because I'm right-handed. This way I could avoid disruption of the port if I decided to throw or break something in frustration.

Going into chemotherapy with the portacatheter saves a cancer patient a lot of grief, especially if treatment persists for an extensive amount of time. I knew I was going to be attached to this medical leash for at least a year, so the day before surgery my friend Mark Wood and I had a field day. We tried to cover a little bit of every sport. It was a six-hour day of playing basketball, golf, throwing the football, and jogging—things I wouldn't be able to do effectively with a central line in my chest (except jogging). It was a reminder that I'd be missing in action for a year. In a way the portacatheter was a relief because my arms and hands would be spared the ongoing intercatheteral abuse.

A week prior to the operation, I was introduced to yet another surgeon, Dr. McElreath. He was from Oklahoma and displayed a southern accent and a very friendly attitude. While waiting for the operation, a couple of the nurses were interested in who was doing my surgery. I said, "Dr. McElreath." They replied in a respectful and convincing tone that he was very good, whatever that meant. I appreciated their vote of confidence.

Surgery involved local anesthesia. The anesthesiologist said I may or may not fall completely asleep. It didn't matter as long as I didn't have to see or feel anything. Sedatives lowered my inhibitions, but overall I was quite alert, talkative, and feeling a little loony. The sight of the surgery was numbed with a butterfly needle while my inhibitions reflected numbness. Dr. McElreath was ready to proceed with the operation minutes after the skin paralysis sunk in. He urged me to express pain if I felt any. When the event commenced, I was in a gown with a sheet over my head and drugged. The images and observations were vague, but the sensations were rather interesting.

I insisted that the doc let me know what he was going to do before he did it. He agreed and proceeded. He said he was making incisions, then I felt the sensation of a scalpel cutting through my upper chest like warm butter. Next, I felt a perception of my skin being picked, as if a little bird was tearing apart a dead carcass. I'd feel subtle gnaws and breaks of flesh as Dr. McElreath cut and sewed the sutures.

The procedure took half an hour. I was coherent and fully alert by the time I settled down at home three hours later. Days later I followed up with Dr. McElreath. My meeting time with him was no longer than ten minutes, but the stipulations that went along with the portacatheter would last for over a year. The top two precautions were to avoid contact sports or any contact in the site area and no strenuous or rapid upper arm movement for my left arm. I was also advised not to lift anything above my head. If the port were to kink or break, the line may be cut off from serving its purpose, thus leading to another surgery to get it fixed or replaced. No, thanks. The line may also slip out of its harbor and cause difficulties. The thing that convinced me most of all was the possibility of the port getting knocked into a lung, and who knows what might happen as a result of that. I didn't want to know nor did I want to risk finding out, not to mention that the half-hour procedure costs nearly seven grand. Compared to the consequences that may result from reckless play, I was more than willing to respect the precautions. I sought compensation by diversifying away from my regular physical activities.

The poison to the cancer in my brain, bone pain, self-injections, sleepless nights, portacatheter implantation, mandatory medications, and all the other miscellaneous grief took place in the first month of chemotherapy. Without loving support, it could have been enough to drive a man insane. I was now living an unthinkable lifestyle; however, I couldn't let the unthinkable control my life. There were other outlets I had yet to discover to compensate for my temporary physical and mental limitations. For the time being, it was one month down, eleven to go, one day at a time.

CHAPTER 8
EVOLUTION

MOM KNOWS BEST

My mom didn't mess around when it came to my diet, especially after the conclusive cancer diagnosis. Everything she cooked was fresh and organic, which was pretty much a staple in her traditional Korean diet.

She read in a Korean periodical that green grapes, without the skin, disrupted the progression of cancer cells and helped to replenish white blood cells. So most every evening or morning during the first week I was back home from OHSU, she'd peel bundles of grapes and throw away the skin. The peeled grapes would then be mixed in a juicer, and poured into a strain so that pure juice, without the pulp, would go into the drinking glass.

Although somewhat tedious, I could see how the process was somewhat therapeutic to wind down after a day at work or church. Either first thing in the morning or some time after dinner I'd drink the magical elixir.

GETTING TO KNOW ME

Sometimes, starting over is the better thing to do. When life flashes before your eyes, perspectives and priorities change. But when life becomes a matter of survival, you are forced you to act and think differently. You are forced to adapt. Losing my short-term memory and ability to recall and translate information was very frustrating. I had no choice but to deal with the circumstances.

Now that I was committed to a year of chemo, there was time to reflect and retrain my brain. Cancer was like a time machine. It seized me in the present, sent me into the past to reflect, then back to the present, and into possibilities of what life would be like if the future was optimistic. During chemotherapy, reflection and perspectives surrounded me on all sides, reminding me of who I really was and how I became that person. Believe me, with no job or school, I had a lot of spare time to think about things—and to conquer video games on my Sony Playstation, including Coolboarders 3 and Medal of Honor.

Thanks to my parents, I have been told that I have an exotic appearance because my dad is Caucasian and my mom is full-blooded Korean. Actually I'm a little German, too, hence the last name of Heinsohn. I even have a sprinkle of Irish in me, notable by the orange goatee hair that I grow. But first of all, let's get one thing straight: My last name is not pronounced *Heenshon, Hensen,* or *Hieenshoon,* but *Heinsohn,* like the ketchup without the 'z'; those damn telemarketers. The *-sohn* is pronounced like *sun,* not *shown* or *sewn.* All together now, *Heinsohn.*

My dad had great taste in music. He owned vinyl from the Doors, the Rolling Stones, Janis Joplin, and the Beatles. As I grew up, he really got me into the Beach Boys; and as the hottest acts debuted new albums, he would buy them, including Michael Jackson's *Thriller,* Bruce Springsteen's *Born in the USA,* and Van Halen's *5150.* We'd listen to Casey Kasem's top-40 countdown every Saturday morning.

We spent a lot of time together over the weekends. During the fall and spring we'd go fishing at Frenchman's Lake for rainbow trout, Pyramid Lake for cutthroat trout, and the Truckee River for German brown trout. Other pastimes we shared included road trips to Oakland to watch the A's. On Sunday mornings we would eat buffet breakfast at a local casino, and afterwards he'd give me a roll of quarters to play arcade games while he played video poker. The Reno Championship Air Races were held in September, and we'd also go on Sunday where the gold unlimited P-51 Mustangs would break world records of over 500 miles per hour.

During the 4th of July weekend until I was a junior in high school, we'd spend seven to ten days at my Uncle Marvin's cabin on Trinity Lake. We'd hike, shoot guns in Uncle Marvin's backyard parcel, and fish for smallmouth bass and rainbow trout. Aunts Marge and Aunt Melva churned homemade vanilla ice cream, and on the evening of 4th of July, we kids would be pyros, lighting sparklers and fountain fireworks for the adults in the family. Aunt Melva and Uncle Marvin were high school tennis coaches, and they taught me the fundamentals at a nearby tennis court. Dad also taught me the simple things like playing catch, changing the oil on a car, and fixing a bicycle flat tire.

The time I spent with my mom was different. She worked at a casino as a blackjack dealer and pit boss. Unfortunately we seldom spent weekends together, since her days off were usually Tuesdays and Wednesdays. Like many first-generation Koreans in the United States, she was deeply rooted in her native culture with a strong work ethic, attention to detail, and pursuit of perfection. When it comes to cooking, she's unparalleled. Her Korean traditional dishes such as bulgogee, chop jay, and seaweed soup were my favorites growing up. She also makes the best home made burritos, crock-pot spaghetti, and baked ham with scalloped potatoes.

Mom taught me how to work with my hands in the arts and crafts. During Christmastime we used to make ornaments and bake Christmas cookies together. She'd prepare the dough, and I would punch shapes with cookie cutters. In the spring, we'd dye and paint Easter eggs together. While my dad was instrumental in keeping me physically active, my mom influenced my creative growth. She was also an exceptional oil painter.

In retrospect I had a happy childhood. I could watch Saturday morning cartoons all day if it wasn't for the fact that they all ended by noon. I got scrapes and bruises from bike and skateboard tumbles. I was famous among my neighborhood friends for my unintentional *endos*, a.k.a., flying over the handlebars and crashing. From time to time I would ride fast down a dirt hill and hit a small obstacle, leaving my front tire stationary as the bike and remainder of my body jolted into the air. I'd walk away with bloodied palms, elbows, and knees. My friends and I liked to catch blue-bellied or horned toad lizards, and I would always try to carry mine home while riding my bike.

My worst adolescent bike wreck occurred when various neighborhood friends and I built a jump in the middle of the street. It was a robust piece of lumber, three feet long. We leaned it onto a Model Dairy milk crate, and it would launch us four to five feet in the air, landing us several feet beyond the jump. The faster we went, the farther we'd go and the higher we'd fly. My first two attempts were moderate, as I landed safely and flat on both tires. Determined to jump higher, I pedaled harder than the previous attempts and soared nearly four feet high, as the front of my bike nosedived on the way down. I failed to pull my handlebars hard enough to compensate for the difference of the previous try.

I endoed hard onto the hot blacktop street, while my bike thrashed and crashed six to eight feet beyond me. The torque left me tumbling, after my hands broke the initial impact with the ground, leaving my hands and knees with enough drag to break through multiple layers of skin. I could see the whitish tissue on the edge of my kneecap as blood ran down my right leg. My leg from the knee down was completely numb, yet I could feel agony if I tried to bend or walk on it. Looking back, I was lucky to walk away without any broken bones. My knee smoldered as I layered water on it, but soon enough, I hobbled my bike back home, six houses down. Even after the wound was washed and disinfected, it was a gooey splotch for days. I limped for over a week.

My first recollection of pain occurred when I was five years old at Uncle Marvin's cabin. I was gathering firewood without gloves, and a splinter became embedded in my thumb. It wasn't pretty, and tweezers would not do the job. A needle was the only way to pry the sucker out, so I was taken outside to a porch where my parents could sit down and work together. I whined and cried whenever the needle poked my thumb. To distract me, Mom and Dad would trick me by saying that Bigfoot was waving at us in the trees. I remember looking up in the trees as they would poke me again and again to attempt to pry the splinter out. Then they said he was going to get me if I didn't behave. They tricked me again and again, until the splinter was out, but I could've sworn I saw a Sasquatch that day.

When I was seven, I got chicken pox. I was almost a week into them, and of course I had to stay home, but that didn't prevent me from riding my bike up and down the block. Somehow I managed to talk my mom into letting me ride with chicken pox. I had them for nearly a week, and they were beginning to scab and fall off. I rode up and down the block at full speed many times. A few hours after the ride, I began to get an excruciating headache. Moments later I thought I was going to die, as my head felt like it was being squeezed in a vice. Mom laid me down on the floor with a cold rag on my head. Minutes later I was at ease.

ROUTINE

Sand in my yearlong hourglass of chemotherapy began to trickle, and my life started to shift into a serious makeover. One moment I'm blazing a trail straight out of college and into a seemingly promising future; the next I am obstructed by a brain tumor diagnosis. Being a cancer patient wasn't the type of lifestyle I had in mind, but unfortunately everyone is eventually dealt a bad hand, right? I was left in the wake of my own aspirations and forced to put my life on hold.

One might wonder what a person with a malignant brain tumor is to do when he is not in the hospital soaking up chemo rat poison. One might also wonder what a patient does when he is not poking himself with necessary injections or taking steroid medications every six hours. For the first month of chemotherapy, I was more occupied with settling into a routine and dealing with all of my protocols. Everything was frustrating and unstructured. I became incredibly agitated, with thoughts surging through my mind like a chicken with its head cut off. Clearly the first month between chemotherapy and my second admission into OHSU was chaos, both medically and mentally. To prevent myself from slipping into complete insanity, I began to read and write. At the time my mind was still in its early stages of rewiring itself into cognitive development. My short-term memory had a long way to go, so the best way for me to rebuild was from the ground up. I began a new journey based on day-in and day-out mental challenges. I had to start over.

Since high school, I have always been goal oriented. When I began chemotherapy, I had no goals, so the first month was like being dropped onto a deserted island. After I was first released from the hospital, I read certain books for therapy and leisure. Other times I documented my medical drama. I had a lot on my mind after my first month of chemotherapy, so I began a more extensive reflection on the past four months of my life. I began to appreciate what I had rather than focus on what I didn't have. I felt immense gratitude toward those who were there for me since the time of my diagnosis, and that's when it hit me: I will write an essay about my unthinkable encounters, emotions, and appreciation for those who were there for me. My friends were my primary source of strength, and I felt they should understand the depth of what I was going through. I began to write an essay.

BACK TO THE OLD DRAWING BOARD

I thought my life was coming together through my five years of college. I explored the world on my own to find out what I like and don't like, and I found out what lies within and beyond my potential; I made mistakes and learned from them; I was adventurous and open-minded. To many this may sound like a person who has his priorities in line, is confident, ambitious, and knows where he is headed in life—someone like myself, I thought. While these are characteristics of thriving on a good life, they evaporate when all of a sudden your life is compromised by cancer. Life became far from cookie-cutter, and my optimism in life all of a sudden turned to skepticism. Whether or not I would go down in flames would now be determined by my medical attention and renewed life perspective.

As an engineering major, I was forced to make sense of the endless combinations of numbers, mathematical equations, science, theory, and various possibilities of solving a problem. The more complex the problem is, the more ways there are of solving it. If I didn't have brain cancer, I was in good health. I was a rare case of a young cancer patient, and the numbers didn't make sense. Without a tumor, the doctors and tests said I was in perfect health for a 23-year-old. I had heard of colon cancer, breast cancer, skin cancer, and prostate cancer, but brain cancer? I'd heard of it, but who in the hell gets brain cancer?

Rather than dwell on uncertainty, I accepted the fact to begin dealing with it. If there was anything positive going through my mind it was that at least the only way I could go from here was up. I couldn't think of anything worse, as my journey through cancer proceeded.

CHAPTER 9

KNOW YOUR ENEMY

The origin of my disease may be accounted for by a number of reasons: life-style, environment, diet, all of the above, none of the above, genetics, or something that was just meant to be. Whatever the cause, there must be some type of pattern beneath it all. Based on my own medical research, I do know that all cancers have one thing in common. According to a number of sources, such as the American Cancer Society, the Leukemia & Lymphoma Society, and Memorial Sloan-Kettering Cancer Center, cancer develops when cells begin to grow out of control from their normal life cycle. Old cells die and new cells replace them, but sometimes a cell may acquire a foreign or genetic change, causing a flaw in its development. Unless the immune system can override the error, the abnormal cell may reproduce over and over until a tumor forms. Eventually, an unsuspecting individual may experience symptoms like headaches, dizziness, or forgetfulness, depending on the location and size of the tumor. CT scans, MRIs, blood tests, and other screenings can help lead to a diagnosis.

My knowledge of cancer and chemotherapy was founded upon firsthand experience. I learned as I went along but later supported my knowledge with printed literature and the Internet. Thanks to years of research and resources accumulated through numerous organizations, doctors, researchers, cancer centers, and universities, I have better understood the nature of my disease.

Exactly why or how cancer cells develop remains unclear, but it seems simple in some cases. Many smokers get lung cancer, some drinkers may get liver cancer, and some people who eat unhealthy foods may get colon cancer. But why or how does a woman get breast cancer, why does a child get leukemia, why do some men get testicular cancer, and why did I get brain cancer? Genetics coupled with environment and lifestyle, perhaps?

The fact of the matter is that, once it happens, it needs to be dealt with. Either that, or it deals with the stricken individual. I was very fortunate to have fallen into the BBBD program, which supplied heavy artillery to attack the cancer, in hopes that it would forever be eradicated from my body. While undergoing the actual BBBD, various chemicals were infused into my brain and into the tumor. From the catheter threaded in my pelvic area to the back of my brain, mannitol sugar solution was infused to open the blood brain barrier. The methotrexate, cyclophosphamide, and etoposide were effective in killing the cancer.

Methotrexate kills cancer cells during the process of their reproduction. Cancer cells reproduce rapidly, so the drug is effective in destroying them. Among potential side effects are changes in skin pigmentation, mouth sores, low blood counts, and possible nausea and vomiting. The skin becomes sensitive to sun, so any changes in the skin must be reported. Mouth sores begin to accumulate like an outbreak of herpes in the mouth if they aren't treated with a simple procedure of rinsing the mouth with water, salt, and baking soda. Other prescribed drugs can aid in the elimination of these sores.

Like other chemo drugs, Etopside interferes with the growth of cancer cells. It may also affect the development of normal cells. Hair loss is the most notable side effect of this drug. I was aware of this side effect, so I was expecting it. I knew it would happen eventually, but when?

The other drug I received was Cytoxan. It also comes in pill form, but that would be an inconvenience, given my regimen. A potential side effect to this drug (along with temporary hair loss) is bladder problems. This drug leaves the body through the urine, so drinking at least eight glasses of water a day is essential. I was fortunate not to suffer any bladder problems as a side effect to Cytoxan.

PROBABLE CAUSES
The Water
When I was a little kid, I developed a habit of chewing ice, especially during

the summer. My childhood friends Jeff Dawson and Josh Wessman will vouch for this. Before and slightly after we were teens, we'd stay up late to watch movies while chewing on ice cubes. About the time I began to play baseball in high school, my mom and dad replaced our old refrigerator with a new Whirlpool. It had an icemaker and cold water faucet that could be accessed from the door. In retrospect the water and ice tasted different but not enough to annoy me. I drank the water and chewed on the ice all the time. During baseball season Mark Wood and I would hang out at my house after school until practice. He sometimes commented that the ice tasted funny and referred to it as "stink ice." While I underwent treatment, I heard from various sources that the lining of refrigerators had residual carcinogens.

I rented the movie *Erin Brochovich* during my time of chemo. The cancer clusters that occurred due to the water from the waste of the surrounding power plants was no coincidence. The same thing happened in Fallon, NV a half our from where I lived. Reports of cancer clusters were reported in the early 2000's among young children from the area.

The Food

In hindsight I consider food in the elementary school system to be a health hazard. At least when I was growing up, our school lunch menus included tater tots, processed meats, canned fruits and vegetables saturated in corn syrup, and artificially flavored fruit drinks.

I could make the argument that the system is flawed by oversights and prevention. Of course in the mid-1980s these health issues weren't relevant to children as much as they are now. I recall one evening I came home from school feeling tired. As day turned to night, I became extremely ill with food poisoning and threw up later that night. It smelled and looked like the breaded beef sticks I ate that day for lunch at the school cafeteria. From that moment on my dad and I called them breaded barf sticks.

The Lifestyle

Thursday, Friday, and Saturday nights in college were full of social opportunities. House parties, beer-drinking games, Greek socials, the nightclub and bar scenes, tailgaters, and college football games. Of course, the majority of those extracurricular activities involved the consumption of alcoholic beverages. I enjoyed and participated in the culture.

As I advanced through college from 1994 to 1999, smoking was allowed in many public facilities, such as bars and nightclubs; in the state of Nevada, anyway. I couldn't stand the thought of smoking but it came with the territory and I just dealt with it. If I could avoid it, I would. But if I was having fun, I tolerated it.

I wouldn't say my diet was much different than that of my peers. If anything, I felt my diet and lifestyle were better than most. Sure, I'd have nightcaps where I'd go to Taco Bell or Jack in the Box to fulfill my appetite at 3 a.m., but so did most of my friends. I also exercised and participated in several intramural sports, along with jogging and mountain biking over the weekend.

I hung around the same social groups and places throughout college, and no one else was ever diagnosed with brain cancer. This leads me to believe that my genetics paired with the environment may have been a contributing factor to my cancer diagnosis.

THE SIGNS
Fall 1997

From personal experience I can testify that brain tumors can hinder a person's way of thinking and feeling. Tumors can cause a person to lose a sense of balance and produce mental blocks of forgetfulness. I recall a few incidences that were symptoms of my tumor. The first unusual sensation occurred during the fall semester of 1997. I was in another array of seemingly endless mind transitions as I sifted through notes, uploaded the computer, and waited for my two lab partners to arrive. It was the middle of the semester, and I was enduring my most time-consuming class, Microprocessor Engineering. The goal of the course was to design and develop a microprocessor system with applications of hardware and software. Understanding the basic concepts of digital electronics was the intention.

As I looked over a board schematic, a strange aura enveloped my senses. My head felt plush and buoyant like a fluffy cloud. Within seconds I lost my sense of sight, as the sensation transformed my vision into a luminous psychedelic pattern of bright tie-dye—perhaps similar to what one would experience in an acid flashback, except I had never dropped acid. Then all the colors merged into one bright light with plasma polka dots. For about ten seconds I couldn't see a thing, regardless of whether my eyes were open or closed. Then, as quickly as it came, it was gone. Sometimes I'd get a head rush from standing up too fast but nothing similar to what I just experienced. I thought to myself, "That was weird," and ignored it as if nothing had happened. Twenty months later, everything happened.

March 1999

The second incident occurred shortly after I returned from my spring break in Hawaii. My roommate Brian Moynihan and I met with some other buddies at a bar to watch our favorite local band, Keyser Soze. Halfway into a Sierra Nevada Pale Ale, I began to feel lightheaded. From lightheaded I became dizzy, and my vision soon began to fade from normal to a fluctuating darkness. I rested my head on my arms face down and realized I was unable to process words out of my mouth. I tapped on Brian's shoulder and mumbled in some indecipherable tongue, intending to say, "Dude. I'm not feeling too good."

He gave me this big grin and chuckled as if I was acting out a facade and replied, "Dude. Are you all right?"

Every time I tried to answer, the words would not come out the way I wanted them to. My head felt as if it were being ripped in a blender. I was swirling, and I didn't know if I was going to pass out or puke. The aura crept up then seized me almost instantly. I didn't tense up, my legs were sturdy, and the rest of my body felt fine. It was my head that was feeling twisted. Slowly, my ability to speak began to process, but I still couldn't articulate normally. I kept my head down and repeatedly mumbled to Brian, "Dude, I'm not feeling so great." I didn't know how to interpret what I was feeling. The sounds in the background were more distorted than a typical night out. They were more like a teacher talking to Charlie Brown saying, "Wa-wah-wa. Wa-wah, wa-wa-wa." The episode persisted for two to three minutes before it finally faded away. I drank a tall glass of water, came to my senses, and felt normal. I continued the rest of the night feeling like myself, but I proceeded with caution.

May 1999

It was three weeks before I found myself in a hospital gown with a brain tumor. I was in an entrepreneur class, where group points are based on team performance, creativity, thoroughness, and quality of work. To solidify my own individual grade of an A, I met with one of the two instructors for a makeup class. There were about 60 students in the class, divided into teams of six or seven. Individual points were based on understanding methods of innovation, venture capitalism, and possible patents. To test my knowledge, Dr. Wang, the professor, asked me, "What is venture capitalism?"

I knew the concept. I knew that it involved making an investment with a chance of considerable financial loss, especially in a startup company. Usually my ability to BS was all I needed to convince someone I understood enough, but in this case, my creativity seemed hindered and next to nothing. I was very inarticulate. Even I couldn't understand what I was trying to say. The first time I was asked, "What is venture capitalism?" I followed with my response. Can't quite remember what it was, but Dr. Wang replied, "Which is . . . ?"

I replied with some jumble of words.

"OK. Meaning . . . ?"

There was silence for about 20 seconds.

"OK. Venture capitalism is blah blah blah . . . etc," Dr. Wang explained once again.

After a second time of explaining, I was asked again, "What is venture capitalism?"

While looking for better words to sound more provocative, I began to explain what I thought venture capitalism was. As words began to spurt from my mouth, I lapsed back into the previous mindset. I was like a scratched record but sounded more disabled every time I skipped. For ten minutes the sequence of questions persisted and reset. My answers were just as mundane as a CD player set on repeat for a track that lasted two minutes. It was horrible, and I couldn't figure out what was wrong with me. "Gee, maybe I don't know what venture capitalism is," I was thinking.

To my surprise Dr. Wang seemed passive from my display of incompetency. I figured it was because the semester was coming to a close, he was busy, and he didn't want to waste his time grilling me. After the incident was over, I graciously thanked Dr. Wang for his time and walked out of the room. My mouth was dry, and I was feeling spaced out. I didn't have a clue.

MONTH II: SEPT 27-OCT 30
Learning the Ropes

Now equipped with the portacatheter, much of any expected agony seemed destined to be over, superficially, anyway. With a portacatheter it's only one poke and all other blood draws and infusions are taken care of through the port. No more human pincushion. An accessed port constitutes my official admission into the hospital. Janeele, the nurse who greeted me into my first preadmission, was now in charge of accessing my port. Like so many other things that seemed to be occurring within the past four months of my life, the unexpected drama *slash* trauma positioned itself to take me by surprise once again.

Before Janeele took me through routine vital checks, she placed two syringes, alcohol pads, Q-tips, tape, and an IV line onto a steel tray next to me. When the vital checks were complete, she requested me to take off my shirt and lie flat on my back. The portacatheter lump in my chest looked like a tumor itself. First she wiped the location of the portacatheter with rubbing alcohol while asking if I was still sensitive from having it surgically implanted. "Not really," I said. She then immersed a Q-tip into a brown liquid called Betadine and smeared it around the port for disinfection. My nerves began to boil once again as she revealed a ¾-inch needle connected to an IV catheter. The pointy object looked like a dart tip, slightly curved at the end, but more like a meat hook in my abstract imagination.

"So how does this work?" I asked.

"I'm just going to stick this directly into the middle of your port. You shouldn't feel much but a little pressure," Janeele replied.

"Sure, that's what a lot of people have been saying lately." I didn't quite buy it. "How do you know the needle will go directly into the portacatheter?"

"The port itself is shaped like a funnel, so the needle has plenty of room to get where it needs to be." Easy for her to say.

Once again, I lay with uncertainty. "Ready?" she urged.

I took a deep breath, "Yeah."

Similar to the surprise when the Foley catheter was first taken out of my groin, I felt a bitter apathy as the meat hook was immersed into my chest. Not that anyone has ever stabbed me, but imagine if someone drilled a hole into the top of your hand. Similar scenario. The pain was instant as the tears rushed down my cheeks. My endorphins instantaneously kicked in once again. I was growing more accustomed to pain, so the pleasure of the aftermath was becoming more exhilarating. I was approaching a point where I almost didn't care. *Thank you, may I have another?*

Spinal taps, Neupogen bone pain, and now portacatheter access. Pick your poison. Personally, if I had to choose, I'd go with the port access. "That was awful," I declared to Janeele. "Is that the way it's going to be every month?"

"Sorry. I didn't think you would be that sensitive," she replied. "There is an ointment called Emla, which is generally applied an hour before a port is accessed." Emla is a cream that numbs the surrounding skin. *Note to self: buy Emla cream.*

Later that day I was scheduled for a neuropsychological exam. I learned that a neuropsychologist addresses the cognitive and psychological behavior of the brain. My neuropsychologist's name was Dr. Paul Guastadisegni, but I had trouble remembering such a tongue-twister. Evidently most of his other patients did, also, so he was suited to being called Dr. Paul. Dr. Paul proceeded to put me through a series of tests, which measured the status of my current abilities. Among the tests were language and verbal skills, visual reasoning, attention and concentration, memory and learning, and motor and sensory function. I was told that the test normally takes between one and four hours to complete. Nearly four hours had passed, and we didn't quite finish. It was decided we'd finish during my next visit.

KEYSER

When I wasn't writing my essay, I was either playing video games on my Sony Playstation, reading, eating, or thinking so much that I began to detach myself from reality. Shortly after I came home from UCLA, and before chemotherapy, Dad threw out the idea of me adopting a dog. He mentioned it a few times before I gave it serious consideration. When I finally showed a keener interest, he laid the responsibility solely on me by saying, "It would be *your* dog. It's *your* responsibility. You take care of it, and you clean up after it." It wasn't like I didn't have enough to worry about. Dad was trying to talk me into doing something he wouldn't take any responsibility for, even though he brought it on. I guess he thought it might be of certain therapeutic value to me. I thought about it a lot and weighed the factors of such things as buying dog food, toys, cleaning up after it, and spending quality time.

Before I departed from Reno for my first session at OHSU, my dad drove us to the humane society, where I scoped out a wide variety of dogs.

There was a boxer mutt with a light brown coat, white paws, and a white tip on his tail. He was the coolest. Unfortunately someone had already placed a holding card to reserve him but only had a week to make a claim. I knew I would be up at OHSU when the card expired, so I signed up as the next person in line to claim him if he was still available.

Shortly after I returned home from my second BBBD and rested for a couple of days, my dad and I went back to the pound. Nobody claimed the dog I was hoping to adopt, so I did. The veterinarian estimated him to be about nine months old and said he was a mix between a boxer and a pit bull. I named him Keyser, as in Keyser Soze from the movie *The Usual Suspects*. My favorite local band was called Keyser Soze, so that's where I got my inspiration.

When I first adopted Keyser, I could see the faint outline of his rib cage because he was so skinny. Within the first month of owning him, he gained ten pounds, weighing in at 61 pounds. Under my care Keyser was a brand-new dog that stood with a more robust posture. He had a lot of obedience to learn, but surprisingly and fortunately he was trained to do his potty business outside. Responding to his new name was a different story, as were certain commands such as *come, sit*, and *stay*. Occasionally he'd get the idea, but most of the time he wanted to play. I didn't mind training, playing, going for walks, or cleaning up after him because, after all, he was my responsibility.

Seven months before my college graduation and diagnosis, my mom and dad moved into a brand-new home, the one I was now occupying. The foundation of the backyard was nicely established with a perfectly green lawn, an automatic sprinkler system, and a decorated concrete patio. Since the house was new, there were no modifications except the hole that my dad dug for a pond liner. The landscape was raw except for areas where the landscapers installed soil. The only existing vegetation was the garden that my mom planted from all the flowers I received when I was at the hospital.

After a couple weeks of Keyser, patches of sod were either peeled off or dragged and mangled, which basically began the day I brought him home. New holes appeared every week, along with patches of dead grass where he peed. Keyser was a one-dog wrecking machine. Because of this, my mom became very upset, and her frustrations infiltrated everyone, me in particular.

I was on very high doses of Decadron, which was effective in treating my tumor; it relieved pressure from my head and was also believed to fight cancer. The side effects, however, were sometimes worse than the chemotherapy. Decadron is a steroid; therefore, it is a stimulant and an inflammatory. My face was bloated, my sleeping patterns were very inconsistent, and my mood swings were sometimes very severe. I could easily succumb to the extreme of any emotion, provided that I had a catalyst. Shit was about to hit the fan.

A dog's a dog, and digging holes is part of a dog's life. I was accepting when it came to cleaning up, feeding, and playing with Keyser. My dad didn't have any problems with him. My mom, on the contrary, became extremely uptight about him, which initiated bad chemistry with everything and everyone. Keyser was destroying the backyard. Every time my mom caught him doing something she didn't like, she would yell at him at the top of her lungs and chase him around the yard. Then she'd come into the house and yell at Dad and I because she wanted a nice yard. This would bring me to a boiling point. Day after day this would happen, and I became extremely aggravated and irritable with everyone. There were a couple of times I couldn't tolerate the yelling, and I shot back with the verbal tone and volume of someone whom I wasn't.

In high school gym class we were educated about the negative adverse affects of steroids, such as extreme mood swings, heightened aggression, heart problems, and high irritability. I would experience those side effects from the Decadron in the months to come and not in the favor of anyone. Combined with a severe lack of sleep, it was as if I could turn into an avatar like the Incredible Hulk in an elevated stressful situation.

HOMEBOUND

Many random occurrences were out of my control and instead were under the care of the doctors and nurses. During the year of treatment, a patient is typically confined to 24 chemotherapy disruptions, two per month on consecutive days. According to MRI scans, which occurred before my second treatment, the remaining tumor was reduced by approximately 80 percent as a result of my first treatment, a tremendous response. It was bittersweet because the chemotherapy was working effectively, yet I suffered a minor seizure. Because it was my first month, the BBBD team decided to limit me to one day of treatment rather than two, to be on the safe side. I hoped to avoid such a complication in the second month. When I woke up from my second passing through BBBD, I felt more relaxed and alert. No seizures occurred, my vision wasn't blurry, nor did I feel so out of it.

After I returned home from OHSU that month, I felt a better sense of control on my raft down the yearlong river of chemotherapy. Let's put it this way, the first month was like trying to maneuver through advanced-class rapids without a paddle or a guide. I had to learn the strokes and behavior of the water the hard way, as I was capsized and banged up against boulders within the white waters of chemotherapy and cancer. But I'm an efficient learner and smart enough to know that fighting the current would only drain my energy and disorient my sense of direction. Instead I learned to ride the tides and use the rapids to take me places.

Because my head was still recovering from craniotomies, it was difficult to hold mindful concentration without straying into la-la land. Reading and writing helped me ease the discomfort but would last for only an hour or two. During the course of the day, I'd give myself shots of Neupogen and Lovenox, take my meds every six hours, pee every hour, and wonder what I could do with myself before going into sensory overload. Dr. Liau, my neurosurgeon from UCLA, gave instructions not to drive for three months after my last craniotomy because of seizure risks. Tolerating treatments well and recovering without unwanted complications helped to convince my dad that

I was OK to drive. I was miserable staying at home, and my parents knew it. A week after returning from OHSU, my dad trusted my judgment and allowed me to drive us both for an errand. I have been driving ever since.

There were occasional instances that spontaneity brought me adventure. It was the first Wednesday of October, and I had been out of the hospital for exactly one week since my second treatment. I awakened, conducted and followed my new ritual of reading for over an hour, and exercised at the gym for two hours. When I returned home, I showered and cooked and ate a hearty breakfast. By the time I was done, it was around noon. I tried to nap but was restless as usual because of the Decadron. I felt the need to get away, but before I left, I made sure to bring water and Extra Strength Tylenol, in case the Neupogen bone pain crept its way into my lower back.

The excursion began with a drive to Donner Pass, off of I-80, nearly 40 miles outside of Reno. I had no plans in particular but to get away from home. When I reached Donner Lake, I proceeded to drive until I arrived at a viewpoint on the opposite side. The weather was absolutely gorgeous that day, so I took a short hike to breathe the fresh air. The next thing I knew, I was driving around the outside perimeter of the lake while listening to Pearl Jam on my CD player. Soon I was at Emerald Bay, approximately 25 miles further. I parked and hiked the nature trail for over an hour. The leaves of the surrounding aspens and black cottonwoods highlighted the surrounding evergreen forest with golden fall colors. I was fond and familiar of the area from when I used to attend summer retreats with my church youth group. I sat on the edge of a boat dock and absorbed the reminiscence for a while.

After my brief rest stop, I continued to drive through South Shore and down Spooner highway until I dropped into Carson City, which was an additional 50 miles. In Carson I stopped for gas at an Arco where a drunken guy had just finished purchasing more alcohol at the counter. He was being a jerk to the cashier as three other customers and I waited for him to shut up and get out. My heart rate began to elevate due to the Decadron steroids. I ignored him as I walked out after I got my change. From Carson I drove home to Reno, as I listened to Creed for another 30 miles. I balled while listening to the song "Inside Us All" over and over again. It was a perfect afternoon that covered nearly 150 miles and six hours. A month later, I added the day to my journal, concluding with: "It's important to make getaways like this often. It reminds me that I am a part of something much bigger, profound, and inspiring."

Unfinished business seems to have a tendency of lingering, and a sense of accomplishment would relieve me of a lot of anxiety. Since I was diagnosed in May, I hadn't accomplished much at my own will because I was too busy treading through shock and the unpredictable. I was, however, reading books, and that was an avenue of accomplishment; but I needed to add a new dimension to my personal therapy, so I set a goal. My essay was on the brink of completion. As a matter of fact, I had enough written material to complete my essay after the first month but decided to hold off until the end of my second treatment, for the sake of thoroughness. The following day, after my return from OHSU, I began to review my previous work and built on it.

Now that I was driving, one thing I absolutely had to do was get back in the gym. I was bored and exceedingly motivated to maintain and increase my fitness. Physically I had done next to nothing for the previous five months, except for walks, and that field day with Mark. I made exercise a mandatory necessity for a number of reasons, including circulation, flushing the chemotherapy out of my system, stimulating endorphins, and venting from being cooped up. Aside from personal medical attention, exercise was priority one.

I enrolled for a membership at a local 24-Hour Fitness, where the manager prorated my membership to a student rate since I was going through chemo. My membership began on October 12.

The portacatheter was implanted on the left side of my chest. I was prohibited from lifting anything above my head with my left arm, especially heavy objects. One of the risks of overextending or applying too much stress on the central line was ripping it out of place. There was a slight stiffness and tug every time I tried to extend my left arm forward. I informed my new trainer, Jake, about my medical accessory and limitations, so we developed a program that would work the same muscle areas but with different ranges of motion. Within a few weeks, between treatments, I was in the gym for two solid hours, six days per week. Day one would be back, lats, biceps, and abs; day two was legs; day three was sit-down chest, triceps, and abs; day four I rested. I'd also incorporate an hour of cardio into my workout.

AN INSPIRATION

One night, when I was watching a *20/20* Barbara Walters special, a guest inspired me. Her name was Liz Murray and she was attending Harvard. She was an exceptional student who grew up in poverty, stayed out of trouble, and claimed that she never touched or abused drugs or alcohol. She was smart. Barbara Walters asked her how she overcame the hard times and resisted the temptation of experimenting with drugs. Liz replied that she preferred to read and make something out of herself. She quoted that "Every challenge in life is a stepping-stone of opportunity."

Long story short, the guest remarked that she used all of her life experiences, good and bad, to become a part of her. She embraced her chaos to learn and deal with her problems. I had the ultimate problem, cancer, and I was dealing with it the best way I knew how by accepting it, staying positive, eating healthier, and surrounding myself with support. I shared my thoughts with Jennifer Enos, and we both agreed that we should deal with our problems before they dealt with us.

SOME FUN . . . FINALLY!

For the first time since March, nearly seven months ago, I was able to attend a concert. Jesse Viner and I were hard-core Pennywise punk rock fans. They performed on October 14 inside the Reno Hilton, but I kept my distance from the thick of the crowd. Until Pennywise performed, I mingled in the beer garden to socialize with a few other friends whom I encountered, but

I didn't drink anything except water. To a certain extent they knew of my condition but didn't know the whole story. Some were mutual friends of Jesse and myself and were genuinely concerned. I was as open to them as they were to me. Others were more superficial but couldn't resist the temptation of asking me.

Pennywise was awesome that night, and it was hard to keep myself from going crazy. Pushing and shoving is a norm at punk rock shows, and sometimes I'd be one to do it in the mosh pit, but my concern was the portacatheter in my chest, and I was careful not to bump into anyone. The energy of the music and the crowd allowed me to distance myself from chemotherapy and release some energy of my own. It was the best time I had since I was diagnosed—a perfect excuse to get out of the house and immerse myself into something I love: music.

THE ESSAY

The following day, October 15, I completed the essay that I had been writing in dedication to my friends and family. It culminated everything I had been through since I was diagnosed up to that point. My fourteen-page, single-spaced composition ended with these statements:

In concluding this essay, regardless of any other trying times, there are some things that simply cannot be denied. Life is right now at this very moment. Life is the privilege of serving hope and promoting well-being. It must be embraced to experience.

CHAPTER 10

ROUTINE

MONTH III: OCTOBER 31 - NOV 27

Admission days of the first four months were the most eventful. Various exams served as a baseline for progress of my cognitive status until I completed my year of chemotherapy. Included in those exams were hearing, visual, and neuropsychological evaluations. As a bonus I was asked to take part in a comprehensive Blood Brain Barrier Disruption (BBBD) patient information video, made exclusively for patients who met the eligibility criteria for the program. It would summarize all the procedures, potential complications, success of the BBBD program, and outcomes. I was among four patients who participated in its filming. The other three were former patients, all women older than forty and in complete remission. Here I was, male, only twenty-three.

Throughout the day a guy by the name of Jim Newman followed me around the hospital with a cameraman, as I went through my various pre-admission procedures and scans. Jim was very cordial. I pretended that the light shining on me from the camera was not there. It was like auditioning for a supporting role in a movie. Jim asked for my thoughts and opinions of the BBBD program, and I replied that it was the best alternative out there to treat my type of tumor. "It definitely gives me hope," I added.

I also completed the remainder of the neuropsych exam with Dr. Paul, which lasted another two hours. When I began taking the exam, Dr. Paul told me I should be done within three to four hours. Instead I was two hours over the norm for a total of six hours between our two sessions. This was evidence that I had a way to go before I could function like I once did prior to my craniotomies. My results, however, were not yet compiled, and I would have to wait another month or so before I received the results.

The following day, Jim was permitted with my consent to shoot footage while I was undergoing chemotherapy. Treatment #3 went as smoothly as the second, and upon my return home, daily shots of Neupogen and Lovenox became a routine, ten- to fifteen-minute procedure. Self-injections became routine. My protocol was to take a dose of Decadron once every six hours. When I reported to Dr. Conrath in Reno, he thought my doses were unusually high for the disease and status of my health. Nevertheless, business is business, and OHSU was taking care of it. The effect was symbiotic; while the pressure in my head subsided, my face became round and bloated. The new appearance made me appear ten to fifteen pounds heavier when in reality I was retaining fluids throughout my body.

CHEMO KINSHIP

Ward 5A at McKinzie Hall became my four-day home during my monthly visits at OHSU. It was where I slept the evening before, during, and after treatment. Ward 5A is where my parents would always say goodbye for the night and where they would be waiting first thing every morning. I'd only be cognizant of 5A before I was underwent treatment on Tuesday mornings and when I woke up Thursday morning.

The patient rooms often slept two, and for the first two months, I didn't know much about the person behind the curtain next to me. I tried sparking conversations whenever I could. One gentleman, who was probably in his early 50s, was very kind and told me of his battle and the support of his family. OHSU was his last resort for a chance at a prolonged life since his body wasn't responding to radiation from his previous regimen at a different hospital.

Often in our conversations he'd say, "Oh Danny, you're going to be fine." I didn't know why at the time but in retrospect I sensed that he knew the end was near. There was just something in his voice. Months later I learned that he didn't make it.

During the first three months of treatment, Monday evenings in Ward 5A were lonely times, especially after my parents left for the evening. Other patients I roomed with weren't social or were already asleep.

On my journey through cancer, I encountered many extraordinary characters who came into my life like guardian angels and saints, including Dr. Linda Liau at UCLA, the BBBD team at OHSU, and Jonathan Yasui. Jonathan and I were a couple of decades apart in age but bonded by brain cancer and two unwavering, loving families. BBBD regimens began at the same time, but we didn't meet until our third month of chemo.

While I was going through my rounds of chemo, my parents would occupy their time by attending support groups, reading, and walking around the OHSU campus. It was there they met Jonathan's wife, Valerie. At the beginning of our fourth month, we would become chemo roommates throughout our treatment regimens. The strength of our families united, and we became each other's best support mechanisms.

Jonathan and Valerie met through a mutual friend in September of 1994. Both resided in Maui, where Jonathan was a journeyman carpenter and lineman who was referred to as the best in his field. Valerie's parents bought her a Hawaiian trip for her graduation present in 1980, and she ended up staying in Maui for 18 years. She had always been in the hospitality business. Valerie brought Jonathan to Portland in December of 1994, where he fell in love with the city. For the first time he could wear a sweatshirt and jeans and not be hot. After they married in 1998, they decided to move back to Portland.

Jonathan's symptoms began with a kaleidoscope vision sensation similar to what I experienced while in computer lab in 1997. Symptoms persisted until one day he received an MRI where they found a tumor in his brain. When the doctor came back with the results he told Jonathan, "Well, you have eight to ten months."

Their world stood still. "What do you mean?" Valerie asked.

"Well, there are three kinds of tumors. 1- you remove and are fine, 2 – there are children's tumors, and 3 – there are bad ones, and that is what you have", the doctor replied.

Jonathan asked, "How do people get brain tumors?"

"It's just bad luck," the doctor said. Jonathan took the papers out of his hands and exclaimed a few choice, colorful words. Valerie's mother was also with them, and they grabbed the X-rays, and left in disgust. In all their lives, they had never seen such horrible bedside manner and lack of empathy. The ride home was solemn and quiet. "What are we going to do?"

The next day a lady from Valerie's medical insurance called and Jon answered. Like Dr. Conrath advised me, she suggested getting a second opinion. And that's when they were introduced to Dr. Neuwelt and Rosemarie. He explained that he had glioblastoma multiform and there is no cure, and life expectancy upon diagnosis was 12 to 20 months. "I cannot cure you but I can give you the best quality of life I can."

Jonathan and I clicked instantly. And instead of waiting around in the hospital or wandering around downtown until our flight home on Thursday evenings, Jonathan and Valerie allowed us to stay at their place. Most of the time Jonathan and I took naps on the couch, or I would sleep in one of their guest bedrooms. Mom and dad would just relax.

RITUAL

Structure to my sanity was maintained by way of everyday routine. During the months between craniotomies I had no structure to support my cognitive mind. Thoughts would take off in one direction and overlap with every other previous idea. Nothing was maintained, as the accumulation of these incomplete thoughts slowly developed into an overlapping pattern of scales on a reptile. Shortly after I came to terms with mortality on earth, my mind shot in one direction: quality of life in the present. Even before my first month of chemotherapy, I had already realized this but not as acutely as when I was diagnosed with cancer.

I was homebound once again. Rather than be spontaneous, it was in my best interest to keep my life simple yet active. The Decadron made my mind race, and if I wasn't busy, I'd begin to merge into sensory overload and become stressed out. Relaxation was hard to come by, unless I had structure in my day; but naturally I was able to be productive with my time. Two of the best lessons I learned in college were time management and planning for the future. Without either, my life seemed overwhelmed. I used those lessons for my daily routine through chemotherapy. Typically I was awake by 6:30 a.m. to start my day. On weekdays I began by picking up where I left off with whichever book I was reading. Although I was still scatterbrained, reading was extremely therapeutic and proved to be instrumental in my cognitive redevelopment. It was an addictive, good way to track my progress from craniotomy trauma.

I'd take my medications every six hours, and depending what time of the month it was, I would give myself shots during the day and include my doses of Leucovorin, which was a mandatory medication to ingest every six hours. Not yet aware of an aspect of simplification, the first week after returning from Portland was still stressful because of my bizarre time schedule for taking medications. The pattern began at ten in the morning on Thursday, the day I was released from OHSU.

I would be given my first oral dose of Leucovorin at 10 a.m. At noon I would have to take my dose of Decadron. Each was to be taken every six hours, so by the time night came, I would be on a very ugly sleeping protocol. Usually I would become tired at ten o'clock in the evening, the time I took leucovorin. Then if I fell asleep, I would have to wake up at midnight to take my dose of Decadron (the stimulant) and Dilantin (the antiseizure medication). If I was lucky, I'd be asleep by 1 or 2 a.m. The alarm clock would ring at 4 a.m. for another dose of leucovorin. At 6 a.m., I would either wake up again or already be awake to take my dose of Decadron. By that time I was wound up again. By 11 a.m. I would give myself routine injections of Neupogen and Lovenox.

It wasn't until after the first week of recovery that things would merge into normalcy. By then I would be off of Leucovorin and daily shots of Neupogen and Lovenox. The only medications I would have to take were

Decadron and Dilantin. Around 9:00 a.m. I'd make myself a hearty breakfast that consisted of either a big bowl of oatmeal with toast or an egg sandwich. If my mom was home, she'd fix me a deluxe omelet. By 11:30 I'd be
at the gym, pumping iron and cleaning out my system with intense cardio.
My workouts lasted for two solid hours, six days a week. I kept to myself
and seldom talked to anyone, but I could always feel eyes looking at my bald
and scarred head.

Stairs led up to the cardio equipment, where I'd begin my workout on
an elliptical machine because it was minimal impact on my legs. I'd do
that for twenty minutes until I burned 200 calories. When I walked down
the stairs, I would have to hold onto the rail because my balance was still
unstable. Sometimes I'd test myself to walk down without the rail, but that
was difficult. I'd count in my head, "one, two, one, two . . . " for each step
because it was easy for me to lose track. If I didn't look where I was going
and lost count, my balance would become unstable, as if I had two left feet.
I'd get confused with which foot should be stepping down. My hand was
never out of gripping range from the rail.

After the elliptical machine, I'd shoot baskets by myself for ten to fifteen minutes before I began resistance training. I couldn't play one-on-one
with anyone because of the portacathter in my chest. The music piped in at
24-Hour began to drive me crazy after my first couple of weeks of working
out. They played the same music day in and day out, with extremely annoying radio hits from Britney Spears and Lou Vega. I recorded my own tapes,
and with headphones I listened to Pennywise, Zebrahead, Rage Against
the Machine, and Filter. This contributed to my introverted nature during
workouts.

To conclude my workout, I'd burn another 400 to 500 calories on cardio equipment. I felt refreshed by the time I was finished. When I returned
home, I showered, read, ate, and took my medications. That was nearly four
hours out of my day, and if I was lucky, I'd manage to fall asleep for 15 to
30 minutes before the racing thoughts from Decadron woke me up again.

From time to time I would vary my routine. By setting weekly goals, I was conveniently flexible, especially without a job. My weekly goals were as follows: workout ten hours/week, practice guitar ten hours/week, write ten hours/week, and read at least one book per month. I drank nearly twenty glasses of water per day to keep my body cleansed. For quite a while I had no interest in TV, but I would watch a couple of shows because they made me laugh. *The Tom Green Show* was on at 10 p.m. Tuesday nights, and *Whose Line Is It Anyway?* was on at 8 p.m. Thursday nights; other than those two shows, I didn't watch much.

Going to movies was a perk of my open schedule because I was under the freedom of my own watch. Since everyone else seemed to have a job or was busy with school, I'd almost always go alone. I didn't mind, because it was peaceful and I was out of the house. Typically, I'd go after my two-hour gym workout, shower, and lunch. Before I left home, I'd called the theater for start and running times so I wouldn't miss any or much of the next movie. At least once a month I would see nothing less than a double feature. After watching the first movie, I would go to the restroom then wander into another theater to watch something else. One day I saw a triple feature. As long as I was back home in time to take my meds, I could watch as many movies as I pleased; or at least until I was caught, which never happened.

SSD BENEFITS

When it came to money, I did not have income. Most of my bills were paid by my diminishing Eurofund—for monthly payments on health insurance, car insurance, and by December, I would have to begin paying off my student loans. I received my Social Security disability application at the end of October, with its endless blank spaces to be filled in to prove my illness. Writing my essay was motivating for me because I enjoyed it, but filing for disability benefits was a nightmare due to my watered down cognitive status.

The paperwork was like outlining a life story, as it grilled me with empty boxes demanding personal information. I was required to list previous employers, type of impairment, liabilities, all miscellaneous and monthly expenses, and friends and family along with contact information. A four-page packet required descriptions of activities, such as the time I get out of bed, sleeping patterns, types of food I eat, chores, odd jobs, quality of life, publications I read, hobbies, and changes in my quality of life, to name a few. The disability report was the biggest pain in the ass because I had to dig out information and dates of all medical-related incidents since I was diagnosed. Cognitively I was only at 50%. I went through my third treatment before I was able to finish the application on November 15.

There are various preexisting conditions that are required in order to obtain these benefits. You must be continually disabled for five months before you are eligible to receive any checks. My timing couldn't be more punctual because I sent my paperwork in on nearly the exact date of five months since I was diagnosed. Once again, I had to play the waiting game until the forces-that-be determined any form of entitlement. Nothing was guaranteed.

KEYSER

On Decadron there was one particular incident that involved Keyser, water plants, and an unreasonable accusation. Before I adopted Keyser, my dad put various water plants into our pond. He bought two water lilies, which cost $25 per pot, and a few other water plant species. The total spent was around $100. Keyser left the plants alone for over a month, until one day my dad looked outside to see him with a water lily hanging from his mouth. The remainder of the pond was empty except for the water. I thought it was quite humorous because, after all, Keyser was just being a dog. My dad, on the other hand, demanded that I clean up all the remnants and replant everything, as if I had done something wrong. "You've got to be kidding," I responded. He responded that he wasn't, and I knew he was serious.

On account of the Decadron I was taking, my severe sleep deprivation, and my father's accusation, I reacted in a way that frightened me. I punched two walls, yelled *FUCK!* at the top of my lungs, and stormed out of the house. My emotions were so intense and I was so upset, it felt as if my heart was about to pound out of my chest.

By the time I walked around the block and returned to the house, I was crying uncontrollably. I hugged my dad, streaming with tears, and said, "I love you."

TIME MACHINE

MY EARLY YEARS WITH MUSIC

While my dad was my main endorser in sports, my mom encouraged me to become involved with music. When I was in second grade, she bought a piano and began to take lessons, in hopes that I would follow. It seems to be somewhat of a trend for second-generation Korean Americans to learn the piano. Most of my U.S.-born Korean friends have mothers who demanded their children learn piano. For months my mom insisted that I take lessons, but I always refused.

I was stubborn, until one day I decided to do it for her. For the first couple of years, I progressed slowly and steadily, with only small interest. My first teacher, Vernita, was retired and instructed me for nearly five years. Week in and week out I would practice the bare minimum, sometimes less, depending on who was watching me.

My mom would get upset and yell if I didn't practice while she and I were at home. I hated being yelled at, but I guess I had it coming. I was wasting time and money for lessons. Sometimes I would bang on the keys to show her how much I didn't like to practice. Other times my teacher would report that I wasn't improving over reasonable periods of time. Countless times, when my mom was off from work, she would patrol the house until I practiced my daily hours or more.

Recitals were trying experiences because I was very shy and nervous when I played in front of an audience. I could feel the heat of my reddening face every time I was the center of attention. For Christmas and fall recitals Vernita would fill her house with several dozen students and family spectators of all ages and skill levels. My best and most memorable recital with Vernita occured in fifth grade when I played the full version of "Für Elise" by Beethoven. I received an amplified applause, and everyone gave me gracious compliments afterwards. My mom was extremely proud, and I felt pretty good about myself, too.

In sixth grade, each person in my class was required to learn a musical instrument. There were two separate classes. One consisted of string instruments, the other of wind instruments, such as trumpets, saxophones, and trombones. The year before, my entire fifth grade class was required to take violin lessons, but when I had the choice to pick an instrument in sixth grade, I chose to play the trumpet, primarily to be with my friends. I continued through middle school and was good enough to play with the advanced band in eighth grade. Most of the brass instruments were guys, and most of the wood instruments were girls. We had the privilege of leaving class early to play at school pep rallies and formal recitals.

In advanced band there were seven trumpet players, all of whom who were determined to obtain first chair. At various times during the school year, each person would be tested to play an assigned song on his or her instrument. The test was better known as a "challenge," to prove who could advance to the highest chair for their instrument at the time. A first chair for any instrument was like a pedestal of excellence. Bragging rights. Throughout the year I fluctuated all over the spectrum from first to worst, but it wasn't until the end that I won first chair. Being last chair was like temporary ostracism. We'd rag on whomever was demoted to last chair. "Hey! How's it going way down there in last chair? Sure is a lot nicer up here at first chair." It was enough frustration to motivate each other to practice harder and attain a higher chair. We had all been down in the pits at one time or another.

Long story short, as the school year progressed, so did the robustness and skill level of my playing. When the end of the school year neared,

I was consistently winning first or second chair. I parted middle school at first chair, but peer pressure and self-esteem issues had gotten the best of me before my freshman year of high school. I didn't want to be considered a band geek, even though I enjoyed playing. My horn-tooting career ended with a very upset and frustrated mom. In retrospect, I can't blame her. Do I regret it? No, but if I was to do it all over again, I would have continued playing throughout high school, perhaps into college. It was all part of growing up and learning from my mistakes.

PIANO MAN

Along with playing in band through middle school, I also continued with piano lessons. I played in numerous recitals. Heck, I even volunteered to play Christmas songs at a church recital with my youth group. At that time in my life, everything was changing, like my voice, my teeth with braces, my self-esteem from peer pressure, and my piano teacher. My mom felt that I was losing motivation to play the piano, so she switched me to a different instructor. Her name was Kathy, and she was much more professional. With Vernita I learned the basics like timing, melody, and finger positions. With Kathy I learned theory and sight-reading. After my once-a-week lesson and before my mom or dad would pick me up, Kathy would put me on the computer to practice exercises for sight-reading and deeper musical concepts. Sight-reading is when you can play a piece of music you've never seen before as if you're reading it out of a book.

Before long, Kathy began to assign me pieces that I would eventually perform in front of a panel of judges. It would be the first and only time that I was judged by a panel (for piano, anyway). Everything else was just recitals. For nearly a year, I practiced four different pieces assigned to me for the *National Piano-Playing Auditions*. There were a variety of pieces that I had to pick from a pool. I chose two classical pieces, "Arabesque" by Burgmüller and "Little Prelude" by Ziooli; and two modern pieces, "Boxcar Rag" by Grove and "Chimes" by Tcherepnin.

There were various ratings for each skill level. Superior was top hon-
ors, followed by Excellent, and I don't remember the other two. It was a
nerve-racking experience, despite the fact that I was able to rehearse days
before in the actual concert hall where the audition took place. I didn't
have to play in front of a big audience, only a panel of three judges. If two
of my three judges rated me as superior then I would have opportunities to
advance to the National Roll, much like an honor roll in school. The audition
was formal, and the students were required to look sharp and present themselves with the proper etiquettes, such as our walk on stage, posture, and
the appropriate bows, according to gender. Boys were suggested to stand
upright, feet together, arms straight on the sides, and a forty-five-degree
bow hinged at the hips. Girls could do the same or step back and bow like a
ballerina if they wore a dress.

Students were to wait outside the of the performance room until it was
their turn to perform in Nightengale Hall at the local university. I was familiar
with the venue, since I performed there with the middle school band earlier
in the year. The performer before me was in the middle of playing his pieces
as I waited anxiously outside the doors. Finally the doors opened, and I
walked in after the previous student walked out, saying, "Good luck," as we
passed each other.

"Thanks," I replied as I began my walk down the aisle towards the main
stage. All I can really remember about my performance was that it went well
except for the two times I hit the wrong notes and froze for a slight moment.
I knew that was a deduction, but how much? A week later, I was commended by my teacher, as she gave me my scores. I received a "Superior
Minus" rating, which meant two judges rated me as "Excellent," while the
other rated me as "Superior." Had I received another superior rating, I would
have been added to the National Roll.

I continued to take lessons until my sophomore year of high school,
a total of nine years. My primary reasons for quitting were because I was
burned out and I wanted to focus my time on competing in high school

sports. I was the only one of all my friends who could play at this level, so I wasn't trying to prove anything. The only reason I continued to play the piano for as long as I did was for my mom.

CHAPTER 11

ENTIRE NEW BALL GAME

DREAMS OF CHEMO

Before I was under general anesthesia during each BBBD, a breathing mask would be lightly placed over my nose and mouth. Sleeping gas would slowly be turned on, and I would be instructed to take in deeper breaths. It smelled like a concoction of plastic and garlic. When the BBBD team was fully prepared, the radiologist would apply pressure to the mask while the gas was increased. I'd be in dreamland within seconds. Once there, a breathing tube would be placed in my throat to monitor and control my breathing.

After my first couple of months of chemo, a strange sensation would form in my mouth. It was like an invisible mass that never took on a constant shape, like a gigantic piece of bubble gum. I'd feel it at random times and in random places, ranging from regular conversation, listening, driving, talking on the phone, or while eating. Then, in my third month of chemo, I began to experience variations of recurring dreams that took place at home in the middle of the night.

Because the portacatheter was in my chest, I trained myself to sleep on my back. I did not want to roll on top of it. One night I awakened on the loveseat at home, feeling as if I was in the middle of swallowing an object. My thoughts nearly paralyzed me as I tried to think of what was heading down my throat and what I could do to stop it. My mind perceived it as a handful of fifty-cent pieces when I came to consciousness. It was like I sleepwalked, picked them up, put them in my mouth, and washed them down with water. Like a visit with the dentist, I didn't want to swallow, but the gag reflex yielded a small amount.

I raised my torso and thought to myself, "You know, I just swallowed two dollars and fifty cents," nearly in a state of panic. "This can't be good." Baffled and paralyzed in disbelief from what I thought just happened, I lay back down to pretend it was nothing; a hospital was the last place I wanted to be. I would rather let the currency pass through my digestive tract and exit a day or two later instead of making a trip to the hospital to get them pumped out. Hours later, I woke up again, and there was nothing ever in my mouth. I pondered the thought often, wondering if I ever did swallow two dollars and fifty cents.

The following month, a similar dream occurred but with a different object. This time it was a double-A Eveready battery. Currency was one thing, but a battery was just plain ridiculous. I got to thinking, "Dude, I just swallowed a battery," but I didn't even move from my bed. "It's too late now." The next thing I figured would happen was the battery acid would start to secrete from the Eveready and dissolve my stomach, then the rest of my body. I dozed off, woke up a few hours later, moved my tongue around, and there was nothing in my mouth. Good thing for me; battery acid might not exit my body as smoothly as a fifty-cent piece.

Another side effect of chemotherapy was mouth sores. A suggested treatment to suppress them was rinsing the mouth with warm water, salt, and baking soda. Sometimes the method was effective; other times, not really. During my ninth or tenth month of chemo, I complained to a nurse on duty of my mouth sores. He offered some lozenges called Mycelex the night before I went into BBBD. They were white, about he size of a nickel, had a bland mint flavor, but they were effective. If only I had known about them earlier.

The nurse who suggested the dissolvable tablets was Steve, the only male nurse I had throughout the course of chemo. I kept the wrapper so I could remember the name in order to place an order when I returned home. A few days after treatment, buying the dissolvable tablets was a priority. I drove to a local Longs Drugs and learned that there was a feminine hygiene product with the exact same name. I asked a customer service person in the women's health care aisles by the pharmacy, "I'm looking for Mycelex to treat mouth sores." She looked at me in disbelief, as if I were some type of freak or prankster.

"Excuse me?" she replied mockingly. Who knows what she was thinking when I asked if they had a yeast infection medication to treat my mouth sores. I had mouth sores that resulted as a side effect of chemotherapy, not an STD. "Come over here and I'll show you what your looking for," as she walked me to the Playtex and Depends aisle. Clearly there was something askew.

I then asked the pharmacist, who replied, "There is, but you have to have a prescription called in for them." I became annoyed with all the BS, so I asked if there was anything else similar to treat mouth sores. The only thing that he could think of was Cepacol sore-throat lozenges. I bought a small package to see if they would work. They were horrible; they made my mouth numb and tasted very bad. I stopped taking them at once and waited until I could get my hands on the proper medication. Nearly a week later, I woke in the middle of the night from another dream in which I had a mouthful of Cepacol lodged in my throat. At that point I simply ignored it and drifted back into a slumber. When I woke up a couple hours later, there was nothing in my mouth.

DATES WITH VAMPIRES

Vampires, phlebotomists, and leeches: what do they all have in common? They suck! So did Mondays.

My monthly admission days into OHSU were Mondays. When I was home to rest and recover, Monday was also a blood test day. Until my year of monthly chemo treatments was complete, every Monday for the three weeks following treatment, my protocol required two kinds of tests: a blood draw to measure my CBC (current blood count) and Dilantin level, and a UA (urine analysis). For the first Thursday of every month after BBBD, another CBC was needed to determine if my body had an adequate white count. If I had a healthy white count after a week of Neupogen, then my body's immune system was robust. If my blood tests told otherwise, I would have to continue with Neupogen self-injections for a full ten days. The end of ten days would be a Monday.

During the two months between craniotomies, I had a few simple blood tests but nothing compared to the ones I tolerated during chemotherapy. Bloodwork was not supposed to be a complicated procedure, but some of the phlebotomists made my life a living hell. In my case, bloodwork consisted of one poke in the arm to withdraw two or three vials of blood, then tape the wound with gauze, a relatively simple procedure. That was a best-case scenario. My protocol from OHSU required four per month. Some of the phlebotomists were friendly, fast, and competent at what they did. I had no problem with the good ones, but I wondered how others attained and maintained their jobs.

Sometimes, when a phlebotomist misses or cannot draw from a vein, another attempt is made on the opposite arm. Other times, the syringe is slightly maneuvered so a successful draw can transpire. Combine a patient whose veins have shrunk from chemotherapy (like myself) with an incompetent phlebotomist, and you get a very upset cancer patient. To get my blood drawn and tested, I went to a lab called Associated Pathology Laboratories (APL). There were a few around town, but initially and for convenience, I attended the one nearest my house. There were a couple particular phlebotomists who were anything but pleasant. I'll refer to them as Cruella and Tormenta.

Cruella was a woman in her late fifties. She was like a witch who was into the art of torture. For the first two months of chemo, Cruella would do most of my blood draws but began to have difficulties because of my shrunken veins. She was never very friendly or cordial. Every time she stuck me with a needle, I felt pain rather than a pinch. On the day that broke the camel's back, she missed my vein on the first attempt and attempted the other arm. When Cruella couldn't draw from the opposite arm, she forcefully manipulated the syringe back and forth, like a joystick. Yet she couldn't get my blood to draw. I thought, "This can't be right," as tears began to melt down my face. It was uncalled-for suffering.

Eventually Cruella succeeded with a small sample, but that was the last time I would ever go to that particular office. After I returned home from that visit, I called the supervising nurse, Barbara, to file a complaint. She said that other patients filed complaints in the past and disciplinary action was taken against Cruella.

Barbara told me of another APL location, which was near St. Mary's. Although the drive was farther, the staff was younger and more upbeat. The new APL was also more crowded, causing longer waits, but there was no way I'd return to Cruella's office. For the first two months there were two phlebotomists who were very competent and nearly the same age as me. They empathized with me and always drew successfully on the first try. Sometimes the office would be understaffed, and I would get stuck with someone new. There was a thin line that separated me from satisfaction and anger, especially because I was on steroids. If someone couldn't get my veins to draw on the first attempt, I would instantly become bitter because I didn't want to get poked twice.

One Monday, a new gal named Tormenta was performing bloodwork. Fortunately she was successful on the first attempt, but I could tell that she was aloof. Some short time later, she was present and attempted to draw my blood again but failed to draw from my right arm. She barely succeeded on the opposite arm, and I began to feel uncomfortable with her because she couldn't look me in the eye. The third and last time I allowed Tormenta to draw, she missed again, then she supported the syringe in my arm and stared at it for almost twenty seconds. I took a deep breath within the long silence and looked down to see that nothing was filling the vial. "So, what's the problem?" I asked.

"It's not drawing," Tormenta answered with a passive voice. There was an inner conflict transpiring inside me because I was trying to be nice about it. I thought, "You're an idiot."

On the opposite arm, Tormenta failed again, as she tried to orientate the syringe by moving it back and forth slowly. It hurt, and I became really cranky. Both arms were now taped and I asked her, "So, now what?"

"We can try the other arm again," she replied. I don't know why, but I let her try again in a vein she previously attempted. I was so ambiguous with my instant mood shifts with the Decadron. Tormenta succeeded, but not before I walked out of the lab infuriated, with my shirt half off. I cursed loudly until I was out of the building. Months and months passed before I ever saw Tormenta in the lab again.

MONTH IV: NOVEMBER 28 – DECEMBER 25
Letting Go

Shortly before my flight for my fourth admission in November, I really began to contemplate whether or not I wanted to continue my responsibility for Keyser. Maybe if I stuck it out for a while longer, things would get better because by now we had spent nearly $600 on him. It would be a shame to let all the time and effort go to waste. I was also starting to get attached to Keyser despite all the grief that he had caused. Sometimes he was a real good dog, others he was a real pain in the ass; but I was on Decadron, which impaired my decision-making abilities. The straw that broke the camel's back occurred one night in early December, shortly after I came home from my fourth month of chemo.

The hour was approaching midnight, and Keyser had to go to the bathroom while I was watching TV. I let him out and closed the door because it was freezing outside. A couple of minutes later I opened the door to let him back in, but he rebelled in a strange manner. He either had bad eyesight or thought I was someone else in the dark because he kept crouching down, staring, and growling at me. Then he would sprint around the yard numerous times. Every time I'd approach him, he would back away, crouch, and run around again. I supposed he was anxious to play. Minutes passed until I finally went back inside with a welcome offer to come along. He did nothing but stare at me. I thought maybe I'll try again in the next half hour to see if he changes his mind. A half hour later I opened the door for a final offer, but he began playing the same game again. I couldn't understand why he wouldn't come inside because it was downright chilly outside.

Sleep was precious, and whenever there was an opportunity to fall into a slumber, I wanted to take advantage of it. With the water lily incident, tearing up the yard, and numerous accounts of waking me up in the middle of the night, I had enough. At this stage of treatment and accumulating sleep deprivation, I made the hard decision to give him back to the animal shelter the next day.

I felt bad, and when I called him the following morning, he slowly trotted out of his doghouse. He looked so innocent, but I couldn't let his charm sucker me. I gathered his food, leash, and toys and loaded them into my truck, feeling a sense of remorse. I almost couldn't do it, but my quality of life would be a lot less stressful without him around. I told my Dad I'd be right back as I walked Keyser out and lifted him into the extended cab of my truck.

When I arrived at the animal shelter, I handed the lady at the front desk my papers and told her I had too many other responsibilities to worry about. There was a friendly African American couple whose faces lit up when I brought Keyser in. I told them he was a great dog and I hated to get rid of him. "His shots are all up to date and has a lot of fun energy in him," I said. The look in their eyes gave me the impression that they might adopt him. I petted and scratched his ears for one last good-bye as he gave me a fat dog lick in the face. He stared in confusion as I walked out the door, and that was the end of Keyser and me.

In retrospect, if I wasn't medicated or my sleeping patterns were normal, I would have the capacity and patience to take care of him. He was a good dog who needed training and the love that I was unable to give him. I tried my best, but my medical situation and emotional leverage were too unstable. In the end it was a relief to let him go. There were other things on my mind, and if I worried about more than one thing at a time, I would become incredibly frustrated. The decision to let go of Keyser was the best for my mom, dad and me.

MOVING ON

A few days after Keyser and I parted ways, some friends and I drove down to Sacramento to see a concert at Arco Arena. The gig was a radio promotion called "Really Big Show" and included some great bands like Pennywise, Foo Fighters, 311, and Incubus. Pennywise is a punk band I had already seen four times, and Foo Fighters is more of a grunge-rock band that I had already seen twice. I am a huge fan of both bands. I hadn't yet seen Incubus or 311 in concert, but Incubus was definitely a must-see for my friends and me. At the time I was pretty neutral about 311; some of my friends liked them, but I had yet to be swayed.

Save Ferris was performing as we walked into ARCO Arena. Upon arrival we didn't think we'd miss any of the bands we wanted to see, but unfortunately Incubus was one of the first acts, and we missed them. Three years prior I saw Metallica at the same venue, Arco Arena in Sacramento, California. A year and a half later, I saw Pearl Jam there. Both were sold-out shows. For "Really Big Show" the venue was barely half full, which surprised but didn't disappoint me. There were plenty of good seats for this general admission show. Usually, when a show promotes numerous big-name, well-known bands, the duration of each act is a half an hour to 45 minutes. The bands in this show were well worth our time. Other than the Pennywise show I saw two months before, this was my second concert during chemotherapy. Once again Pennywise was great, but what I appreciated even more about their performance was that they played a cover song by Sublime called "Same in the End." I love Sublime, but I never got the opportunity to watch them because of front man Bradley Nowell's untimely passing.

Foo Fighters were next, and the experience was completely different from the other two shows I had seen them perform. I was almost a hundred yards away when I saw them at the Tibetan Freedom Concert in 1996. A year and a half later, they performed at the College Greek Ski Weekend in Reno. I was intoxicated and in the mosh pit the entire show. Now that I was attending my second concert during chemotherapy, I was comfortably numb with a relaxed and excellent view of the band. It seemed surreal compared to the first two times I saw them. 311 performed next. I didn't know what to expect of them, although I listened to and enjoyed one of their albums, *Transistor*. I was highly impressed with their show as they performed an energized, eclectic variety of hip-hop, funk, rock, and reggae. So far (and by far), live music gave me the most joy during my time of chemo.

CHAPTER 12

PHASE SHIFT

MONTH V: DEC 26 – JAN 23
Neuropsych Results

Christmas and New Year's straddled my fifth month of chemo. Due to prior time constraints, I didn't receive hard copy results of my neuropsychology exam from Dr. Paul until the day after Christmas. The results were insightful but not surprising that I was in the average to below average range for intellectual abilities. The problems most relevant were those that resulted from my first craniotomies back in May 1999. Speed of information processing, short-term memory, and working memory were noted as below average. I knew I progressed a little from my first surgeries, but I didn't know the deficit until this point.

My memory function was most impacted when working with auditory and verbal information. I could only handle one thing at a time. Dr. Paul stated that my capacity to do multitask chores and shift back and forth between information was limited. I asked him to give me an example. He replied I would have trouble with something like talking on the phone, cooking, watching the television, and taking a message. He was right. My attention span would stray into a senile state if I was the least bit distracted.

My scores were consistently low with my attention span and slow when processing auditory and verbal information. My ability to hold an interesting and engaging conversation was flawed, although verbal fluency was something I noticed improvement in as the months wore on from first diagnosis. I could process bits and pieces of a concept, but my ability to comprehend was like absorbing Silly Putty into a sponge, especially with more complex information. If a college professor were to ask me to summarize a lecture, I would fail because responding with articulate feedback was difficult. Doctor Paul's evaluation stated: "He is experiencing a change in his cognitive abilities, which appear directly related to his tumor."

The strengths I possessed resided within visual reasoning, where I achieved average to superior ratings. My ability to arrange patterns and identify differences in pictures were rated particularly high. Dr. Paul suggested I get into a routine, keep things simple, and don't overload on information. A change in routine and a lack of structure could contribute to confusion and difficulty in functioning. I was encouraged to increase my daily activity as long I could maintain a threshold without becoming confused and frustrated. Frustration was part of the recovery process. Coincidently, everything suggested was already initiated from my own motivation.

Y2K

Y2K was rather uneventful and depressing. I returned from my fifth month of chemo on the evening of December 29th. My friends threw a New Year's bash that I really wanted to attend, but two days' rest after chemo wasn't enough time to for my immune system to recover. Instead I watched other prerecorded, televised New Year's celebrations from around the world. The world didn't end, and the Y2K bug didn't crash all of the world's computers. I was safe at home with my family, watching the mesmerizing fireworks shows from around the world. The Eiffel Tower in France and the bridge in Sydney, Australia, were among the best New Year's spectacles I had ever seen.

THE TUNNEL

Around my fourth month of BBBD, Rosemarie told me about a guy named Ryan Hutton who once had the same disease as me, and she thought it might be therapeutic to get in touch with him. Weeks following, I received an e-mail from Ryan, which stated:

Rosemarie asked me to contact you regarding your treatments. Like you, during 1993–94 I went through the same treatments you are doing. She thought perhaps you would like to talk to someone close to your age and what it was like etc.

Finally, someone I could relate to. I responded. Nearly two weeks after New Year's 2000, I received a response from Ryan on January 12, which stated:

I'm glad that you wrote back and hope you had a great New Year's. I have yet to read your essay, as I wanted to get a quick reply to you. I will be turning 32 this Jan. 18. I was 25 when I was diagnosed with primary CNS lymphoma. A doctor told me that I wouldn't live past 18–24 months. Even if I die tomorrow, I will be happy knowing that I outlived his prediction. I had a total of 24 treatments in 13 months, the reason being that one month I got only one treatment and later down the line I got only one. So at the end I insisted that I get another month to complete the 24.

At the time of my diagnosis, I was in my second year of law school. After I completed my treatments in March '95, I went back to school and finished. I soon after took the bar and have never looked back. So far my scans are clean; only God knows what the rest of my life shall entail. However, thanks to him and Dr. Neuwelt, I have had six years that I never would have had. I feel that I've lived a lifetime in those six years and hopefully will keep on.

In parting, I will share with you an analogy that I used when I was asked what it was like to go through these treatments. I'm sure you can relate. When you are told that you have cancer, it is like someone throwing you into a deep dark tunnel. You are frightened and scared and unsure of what to do or think or act. Doctors come along and point the way, way down the tunnel and say: "You see that faint light? That is

your salvation and we are going to help you get there." The doctors then
proceed to take out baseball bats and beat the crap out of you. They pick
you up and tell you to keep walking towards the end of the tunnel. "We
will meet you farther down," they say. You walk and you see them, and
again they beat you with baseball bats. As you get closer to the end, it
gets harder and harder to get up and keep walking towards the light.

> *Just keep walking, it's worth it.*
> *Take care,*
> *JRH*

The analogy was vivid, and I was taken aback in tears. I was nearly
halfway to the end of my journey, and in this moment I felt great strength.
I knew I would be a survivor. Ryan's words were beyond comforting and
inspired me to write in my journal.

JOURNAL ENTRY
1/18/01

It's amazing what can be discovered and learned through the course of our lives.
It baffles me to know what some people are led to believe. It's understandable
though, that some people believe in certain things because they are either misled
or afraid. So afraid that they wouldn't know how rewarding life could be if they
just got up and took control of their life. Having the foresight to live out a dream
on your own terms is truly a privilege to the nth degree.

As I have been walking down this newly paved path in my life, I have dis-
covered and seen many new perspectives and truths. In fact lately I have been
experiencing a phenomenon that I cannot yet explain or describe consistently. I
may never. Somehow I understand it. I feel as though this phenomenon has been
deeply conforming with my life and becoming a part of me. I accept it with all
my heart. As it evolves and grows, I learn more about myself, and my life becomes
more spiritual and indescribably profound with meaning. According to the way
I've seen society work, I feel I have been given this phenomenon as a gift. At my

age or generation, how many people get to truly discover what they are made of? On that conviction, how many people even get a chance to put themselves up to that challenge?

When the chance to try something new presents itself, seize it, especially if it's something you've dreamed of doing. Be prepared for those opportunities, but don't expect them to go as planned. Be ready for excitement. Realize that the path we choose in life is always changing, and that is what keeps us on our toes.

TIME MACHINE

COLLEGE: THE FIRST FRONTIER

Upon graduating high school, I didn't have a clear direction as to what I wanted to do in life. Our senior trip was in Mazatlan, Mexico, and I had the time of my life. Out of 387 of my classmates who graduated, nearly 100 of us had one of the best weeks of our lives. My aspirations of playing college baseball died after a disappointing senior season, but when I returned from Mazatlan, my outlook on life changed. I didn't quite know what I wanted to do, but I wanted to have fun along the way.

When I was in grade school, I was a big fan of Superman. My mom and dad would take me to the movies, and I was always so inspired when Christopher Reeves saved the world. I loved the soundtrack, the villains, and the heroics. Eventually reality set in, and there were new influences from family, youth group, and school.

As I grew up through adolescence, I expressed my creativity through drawing pictures. I was always one of the most recognized artists in elementary school. In fifth grade I won a poster contest that awarded me fifty bucks and a formal breakfast with the governor and other state officials. The contest was to draw a picture that represented what freedom meant to me. I drew a collage of a bald eagle, the White House, the U.S. Constitution, the American flag, the Congressional Medal of Honor, a cannon, and other little icons that represented freedom to me. Along with a few other students from the district, we all shared the privilege.

At the breakfast we were required to give brief presentations of what our posters meant. I was painfully shy, nervous, and anxious to get out of the center of attention. Prior to that recognition the first thing I remember winning independently was a Halloween picture contest in second grade. I won a coupon for a free Round Table pizza.

Relatives would hear about my success in the poster contest, winning spelling bees, or whatever else family and relatives like to brag about. Those milestones occurred when I was entering my teens, and UNLV was a big name in college basketball. I was a huge fan. At the time in the early 1990s, UNLV had a respectable school of architecture, and that's when I began to think about what I might want to do in the future. I filed those aspirations in the back of my head as I entered high school. Eventually I became disinterested because I got sidetracked with varsity sports.

When I realized that playing baseball wasn't meant for me, I explored my options through past inspirations. The main reason I was driven to declare civil engineering as a major in college was because of my youth group leader in middle school. I looked up to him as a role model, and he was studying civil engineering while in college.

I concluded that life as an engineer would allow me to be financially comfortable, so I could afford the other activities I wanted to do in life. It seemed inevitable that I would work most of my life, so I may as well make good money doing it. That was my perception back then.

I was on the five-year plan in college, and by the time I graduated, I changed my major three times. After my first semester of civil engineering, I didn't like the thought of being the person responsible if a structure I built collapsed. But I had a few more semesters to figure out what I wanted to major in. I tried accounting 101 my sophomore year, and it bored me to death. Mechanical engineering was a thought until I took statics in summer school while working full time. I was out of my league and barely squeezed by.

By the time I finished my core classes of physics I, II, and III; calculus I, II, and III; and differential equations, I had fared rather well in these electrical engineering prerequisites. I sailed through my last two years with a 3.0 average in the college of electrical engineering while staying actively involved in extracurricular activities, volunteer work, and holding down a part-time job.

Throughout my five-year tenure at the University of Nevada-Reno, I worked for seven different employers. My first job before my freshman year was a loader for UPS, which didn't leave much time for a social life after an evening shift. To become more socially involved on campus, I took on a different job at Long's Drugs, where I worked as a cashier, warehouse stocker, and customer service representative for six months. After Long's I found a job with more flexibility and higher pay at Arrow Electronics, which was a Fortune 500 company.

Arrow Electronics was a distribution center for electronic components and equipment for corporations, such as Intel, Hewlett Packard, and Texas Instruments. Although my job became mundane at times, days went by fast. The best incentive for working at Arrow was the flexibility it offered part-time employees like myself. As long as I worked the minimum of twenty hours per week, my boss was flexible with my busy college schedule.

The Reno branch consisted of approximately seventy employees, and a handful were fellow part-timers. My job title was picker, and my duties were to pick out orders through designated aisles, count the parts, place them into an electrostatic safe bag, seal the bag, scan the label, and move to the next order. When I completed a batch of job orders, I'd send them on a conveyer belt for packaging and shipping.

Job performance was based on quality. In my department the average picking error per person was two per month. I worked for seven months without one error, and upon completion of my first year, I received employee of the month recognition. I obtained the privilege of the VIP parking spot and a lunch at the restaurant of my choice with the company managers. My boss also felt that I deserved the raise I had been bothering him about during the previous months.

I was halfway through my college career during my time with Arrow Electronics when I began looking for internship opportunities on campus. I became involved with the local chapter of the Institute for Electronic and Electrical Engineers (IEEE) and volunteered to help the president and vice president with some of their marketing efforts. I made phone calls and posted flyers around campus to promote the organization. I asked the president if she knew of any companies in the field who were hiring interns for the upcoming summer, and she gave me an application for the company she was working for, Sierra Pacific Power Company (SPPCo).

Within a week after I submitted the application, I was called for an interview and soon offered a position to work as an intern in their telecommunications department. I accepted. Two weeks later I was offered an intern position with gaming machine manufacturer IGT, which was my first choice; but I declined it, since I accepted a position with SPPCo.

My internship for SPPCo would last for a year. Within that time I updated over a two years' backlog of CAD files, learned the ins and outs of the utilities power grid, and designed the department website. I was also assigned a project coordinator role to license and implement a frequency with the FCC for an alarm system at the local water treatment facilities.

The following year I worked with one of the professors to develop a campus parking meter system that would increase parking revenue. It wasn't popular among my peers because any residual funds left on a meter would automatically default to zero once the paying vehicle left.

Finally, during my last semester, I interned for Hamilton Company to develop circuits that allowed project managers to test fluid precision instruments before delivering them to hospitals, doctors, and pharmaceutical reps. In other words any medical syringe or vial that contained therapeutic agents for my treatment was probably a byproduct of Hamilton Company. Who would've thought I'd be on the receiving end not long afterward?

CHAPTER 13

REALIZATION

MONTH VI: JANUARY 24 – FEBRUARY 20
It's My Party, and I'm Going to Have My Cake

I am an only child, and one thing my parents knew how to do really well was throw a great birthday party. In my pre-adolescent years I invited my closest friends for parties at Chuck E. Cheese or Show Biz Pizza. As I grew into adolescence, I'd throw slumber parties, and we'd go bowling instead of playing games at arcades. My mom would always bake cakes and decorate them with different themes each year: baseball diamonds, space scenes with astronauts, or winter scenes with trees and skiers.

While in elementary school my dad would rent horror movies for us kids and take us to Baskin-Robbins for ice cream during slumber parties. When I got my Nintendo one Christmas, everyone would take turns playing in the guest room. The following morning my dad would always cook pancakes of various sizes and bacon, while my friends would take turns playing new Nintendo games.

On January 27, I returned home from OHSU and was officially halfway through my year of chemo. Before I went to OHSU for my sixth treatment, my mom asked what I wanted to do for my 24th birthday. She wanted it to be special, but I was adamant about it being nothing elaborate. At the very most, dinner with a few friends was good enough for me, but Mom persisted in throwing a party. The more she asked and suggested, the more motivated I became. I began calling people on Wednesday for a party I would throw two days later on Friday.

Ever since I began chemotherapy, and from time to time, Jesse Viner and I would jam on our guitars. We practiced many songs together but most often played "Nutshell" by Alice in Chains, "Badfish" by Sublime, and "Everlong" by Foo Fighters. Since the party was such a last minute, we had only one day to prepare our show night. Although rusty, we were good enough.

I felt like a kid again. I was kept constantly busy in thought and preparation on the day of the party. Mom prepared sushi rolls, and I ordered all the other food and beverages. I called my friends on Wednesday and told them my party started at 7 p.m. Most of my guests knew each other in one way or another. My friend Jon Pabico was the first to show up at 7:30. Jon is an amazing piano player, and everyone marveled at his talent. Coincidently he was the last to leave at 2 a.m.

Jesse and I played our three songs, and I sang. It was after 9:30. By that time there were around 20 people, mostly close friends. I felt incredibly humbled to have them support me through the tough times. After Jesse and I completed our set of three songs, I played a solo of "Elderly Woman Behind the Counter in a Small Town" by Pearl Jam. I was almost emotional when I finished. Everybody gave Jesse and I a gracious round of applause, and it was one of our finest moments.

Guests showed up in random intervals and stayed for different durations, but when all was said and done, a total of 31 people attended. Most of my guests didn't think I would have much food, yet there was enough extra to serve at least ten more people. I felt a little guilty because I thought my house would be too crowded, so I limited my invites.

Sunday, the day after my actual birthday, Jennifer Enos and I attended the infamous street band ensemble show *Stomp*, performed in rhythmic harmony using unconventional percussion instruments, such as oil drums and dustbins. It was a highly captivating show.

A WORD FROM UCLA
Dr. Linda Liau, my neurosurgeon from UCLA, had this to say in response to my essay, "Regarding Hope," on February 14:

Hi Danny,

So glad you're doing well. Having patients like you is very inspiring to a neurosurgeon. I have another patient who's only a few years older than you with a malignant brain tumor. She's really having a hard time dealing with it. Like yourself, she had just graduated from college (UCLA) when she first learned about her disease.

Would you be willing to share your story with her? I think it might help her . . . if so, I'll give you her address so you can write to her.

Keep in touch,

Linda Liau

I was flattered by Dr. Liau's feedback and my desire to become a writer, inspire, and teach was affirmed. February was the sixth month and midway point on my long road of chemotherapy. I couldn't wait to finish the journey. The rest of my life had finally caught up with me, and a radical transformation had taken place. I was a new person with a new perspective and motivation to chase my dreams and help others.

TIME MACHINE

WORK ETHIC

I had a strong, disciplined work ethic when it came to high school sports, particularly baseball. And there wasn't much I wanted to do during the summer before my senior year but play summer ball. I was passionate, there was no pressure, and it was the best summer I had playing the game. I got ample playing time and was sometimes relieved on days we didn't have to play, although I wouldn't have minded if we did. The team was comprised of returning seniors and some good junior prospects, many of whom I grew up with while playing Little League.

It was a loose season, and we had fun playing the game. Of course it mattered if we won or lost, but no one cared much about keeping score until it was time to pursue another state championship. By the time school started, I was at the top of my game, with a batting average just under .500. I hit at least one double in each game for our last ten games. I had good speed, legitimate power, and consistency with the glove at third base. My pitching was on the mark, as I chalked a few gems under my belt.

At the end of that summer, before my senior year in high school, I really wanted to play baseball in college. I lived and breathed baseball. My room was wallpapered with baseball posters, magazine clippings, and pennants, a third of which was Bo Jackson, who was my all-time favorite athlete. He could do it all until his hip was dislocated when he was tackled while playing Tampa Bay in 1991. I remember it vividly and was stunned when I saw it happen live on TV. After replacement surgery and recovery, he returned to baseball for the Chicago White Sox and hit a home run in his first at bat. I was inspired by his comeback.

I played varsity tennis in the fall season during my senior year along with Mark Wood and Todd Russell. Todd and were I on the same Little League all-star team. We played doubles and maintained first seeds throughout the season, while Mark was the staple for our number one singles seed. Most of the competition was above our level, but we gave a lot of the top schools a run for their money and held a winning record in the end.

When tennis season ended, I went right back into baseball training for the winter months. I spent countless hours in the batting cages, facing a pitching machine that was four feet closer than the regulation distance of 60 feet, 6 inches. At that range I was consistently driving balls on the 80–85-miles-per-hour machine. By the time spring came along, my timing was all screwed up.

I also spent a lot of time in the weight room during the evening on weekdays. By the time the season started, I weighed nearly 170 pounds and could bench press 215 pounds. While the close proximity of the pitching machine screwed up my timing for hitting, lifting weights screwed up my pitching mechanics. I wasn't able to redeem myself in either discipline and

saw a lot of bench time. My running speed and fielding were my only reli-
able assets to the team, so I would be the go-to pinch runner in any critical
situation.

While my baseball career didn't go as planned, I still loved the game
and took with me all the lessons it taught me along the way, including a
strong focused work ethic. I still had an unwavering desire to be successful,
and I always strived for excellence throughout college. The Pi Kappa Alpha
fraternity exercised strong core values, such as integrity, leadership, team-
work, etiquette, and being gentlemen.

I brought my work ethic to the college campus and held various chairman positions through the fraternity, including campus activities, fundraising, social, and brotherhood roles.

Our chapter held an annual fund drive event called the Sorority Bowl,
which was a one-day bracket tournament among all four sororities on campus. The beneficiary was the Committee to Aid Abused Women (CAAW).
My job was to coordinate the entire event, which included all marketing initiatives, sponsorship renewals, branding, PR, and frequently meeting with
the sororities. Yeah, tough job, but someone's gotta do it.

I renewed all of our current in-kind sponsorships, which included sandwiches, pizza, nonalcoholic drinks, printing services, and award medals. I
leaned on the past chairman to help me put everything together. For the
brand theme of the event, it was decided to use the Heisman Trophy and
have a professional artist superimpose a woman's face on the trophy. That
branding theme went on all the T-shirts we sold and on the Sorority Bowl
event programs, which were distributed during the week before the game.

A week following Sorority Bowl was homecoming. It was my responsibility to inform the actives what events were happening and when. My prime
obligation was to ensure the float was successfully under construction and
completed by the day of homecoming. This meant meeting with Pi Phi's (the
sorority we were paired with) to work on the float together in the evenings.
At least I wouldn't be in this one alone. Homecoming represented campus

pride, which meant Greek pride, which meant sorority pride, which meant participation, which meant everyone was obligated to contribute.

When the Friday night eve of homecoming had arrived, the float was on the verge of completion, and it was the pledges' job to fill in any unfinished sections and stand guard overnight. Sabotage by other rival fraternities was likely. I hitched it to another Pike's full-sized Chevy Blazer so it would be ready for me to drive in the morning. I came home around eleven o'clock that night and managed to look over some homework.

The following morning I was up by six; I didn't shower, just ate breakfast and scooted my ass over to the Pike house. By the time I arrived, everyone had retired from the long night. A pledge named Rich remained. He was the chosen one who would ride with me in the homecoming parade. Nearly an hour before the festivities, we arrived, parked, and waited at the beginning of the strip, as sororities, fraternities, and other social organizations rendezvoused around the same area.

The week was long and sleep-deprived, but the final results made everything worthwhile. There were over a dozen cute Pi Phi's who rode our blob of chicken wire and napkins. I drove the pride of Nevada down the strip while thousands of people cheered and waved at our float. I felt really good about what I was able to accomplish that semester, even though my grades suffered.

I learned two valuable lessons that semester. One, approach large projects with a plan; and two, become efficient with time management. My strengths and weaknesses had been exposed through chaos, but in the end I evolved into a higher state of self-awareness for problem solving. My fall semester GPA was reduced to a 1.67 but I bounced back with a 3.3 GPA in the spring.

CHAPTER 14

A NEW BEGINNING

THE NEXT THREE MONTHS

During the first six months of chemo, it seemed I experienced the extremes of all my emotions: shock, bliss, frustration, fright, anger, sadness, loneliness, exhilaration. During the next three months, nothing stimulating happened. Anxiety and complacency began to infiltrate my mental composure, along with the mainstay of Decadron, which continued to amplify my moods. My wave of introspection and reflection within my downtime was beginning to dissipate, and I began to feel a sense of isolation. More than ever I became anxious about going into remission and moving on with my life. The weather began to warm up, and I became somber because I longed for regular outdoor activities in the sun. I was bored with my monthly gym routine, and I lost my motivation to attend regularly. My pace of reading two or three books a month was reduced to one a month.

MONTH VII: FEBRUARY 21 – MARCH 21

The Leukemia & Lymphoma Society

At the beginning of March 2000, the Leukemia & Lymphoma Society of America (LLS) found me, likely from doctor referrals. The initial contact was a letter offering reimbursements to qualified patients for medications, travel, and other expenses. I was informed of the organization's patient-support groups and seminars about living through cancer and chemotherapy. By this time I dwelled in my own, well-earned comfort zone but was open to discussion and contribution regarding my illness and related ones.

A patient's rights forum was held in Sacramento in mid-March, where my Dad and I drove to learn more about it. Most who attended were proactive patients or survivors, open to sharing and contributing in the fight against blood-related cancers. Unless told otherwise, one would never know of their diagnoses—unlike me, bald and with a horseshoe scar on the side of my head. Patients share the same equal rights as any American citizen. They are to be treated with dignity, respect, and not to be discriminated against because of a diagnosis. Most important, survivors and patients have the right to pursue happiness.

Back in Reno a couple of weeks later, the LLS arranged for me to meet with a leukemia patient close to my age. His name was Jeff Cooney, and he was the first person I met of my generation with a blood-related cancer. Although the nature of our diseases and treatments were completely different, we bonded through our ages and stories. Jeff was diagnosed with acute lymphocytic leukemia (ALL) two weeks after I began chemo. Immediately after diagnosis he began seeing Dr. Conrath, who referred him to a specialist at UCSF, where he then underwent a stem cell transplant in January.

Jeff's passion was golf. We shared other common interests, such as mountain biking and traveling. We met at a café in a tennis club, and he was accompanied by his girlfriend, Minette. A couple of affiliates from the Sacramento chapter, whom I met weeks earlier, organized the luncheon and they also attended. Mom and Dad escorted me and sat in with us. The primary purpose of the rendezvous was to introduce Jeff and me to the Leukemia & Lymphoma Society's *Team in Training* (TNT). Our stories would be the currency for endurance athletes to train for marathons and 100 mile century bike rides while raising money for the cause.

Jeff also became friends with one of my fraternity brothers, Curtis Fuestch. Curtis was a senior in college when I was freshman at UNR. Through Jeff I learned that Curtis was living with leukemia as well. The bonds were mutual, and Curtis was making his way in life with minimal treatment and side effects by that time.

MONTH VIII: MARCH 22 - APRIL 16
New Roots

Team in Training was the primary fundraising arm of the Leukemia & Lymphoma Society. Participants of *Team in Training* raised millions of dollars every year by way of training for an endurance event. Over the course of four to five months, each participant would be obligated to raise a certain amount of money dedicated to someone stricken by leukemia or lymphoma. The goal event would be a marathon, century (100-mile) bike ride, or triathlon. Anyone can join, with the intention of being part of a team, commitment, and mission to raise funds towards the battle against blood-related cancers.

Due to my condition I was naturally inclined to become involved and had no problem making a personal connection to anyone dedicated to help the cause. In fact I was the one who felt honored to be recognized and represented. Honorees were invited to various events, parties, fundraisers, and team workout sessions throughout the training season. Within that time, the team is obligated to raise money on behalf of an honored patient. When a TNT participant raises a certain amount of money, he or she is automatically enrolled into an all-expenses-paid trip, which includes airfare, hotel accommodations, and meals to wherever their target event takes place. San Diego, Sacramento, and Lake Tahoe were a few of the primary destinations at the time.

The awareness of LLS in Reno wasn't as exclusive as I thought when I was inducted as an honoree. There were less than twenty who participated at the close of my year in chemotherapy. I was represented by two lovely ladies in their early thirties, Kelly and Veronica. I only became acquainted with Kelly through a lunch rendezvous. Because she was running for me, I shared my story with her. As I perceived it, many people who participate in the LLS *Team in Training* program do so because it's for a good cause; but they aren't really connected to the actual reality unless a personal connection is made with a patient. Most patients seemed to be children who weren't yet cognizant enough to realize the true nature of their illness and the impact made on their families.

I told Kelly what I had been through and that I was writing a book about my journey through cancer. Like myself she was in the process of writing a book, but she wasn't yet persistent enough to follow through. We agreed that writing a book is quite a task. During the course of conversation I mentioned that I played the guitar. She replied that her husband also enjoyed playing the guitar and regarded him as very talented. "He plays the most incredible songs from the top of his head," she says. But like me, when asked to play the same song again, he doesn't remember because everything he plays is whatever comes to his mind at the moment. She mentioned that, if I ever wanted to jam with him, she could probably hook us up. Also, if I needed a critique on my writing, she said she'd be happy to do that as well. Lunch with Kelly was pleasant, but that was the last time I talked to her, even after the marathon she ran in Sacramento on December 3, 2000.

My blood counts were on the low end of borderline that month; in other words the doctors required another blood test before I could be admitted to OHSU. Rather than be admitted on the usual Monday, I had to wait until Wednesday. Although the delay was only for two days, I was frustrated by the inconvenience, mainly because the synchronicity of Jonathan's and my routine was broken. He tolerated the BBBD better than me because he never had seizures while undergoing treatment. He was also always more alert when leaving the hospital.

During that offset seventh month I should have been out of the hospital and back home on Saturday, but there was a new nurse who I thought was rather cute. She tended to me in the wee hours of the morning but forgot to administer my mandatory IV dose of Leucovorin at four in the morning. Before I was sent home, someone from the nursing staff realized the mishap, and I was not permitted to leave the hospital that following evening. Rose Marie said that the dose was crucial, and the toxic effects of the chemo could be severe if it wasn't neutralized. The nurse responsible for the mistake was written up, and that was the last time I saw her. I was upset because her mistake grounded me in the hospital for an extra night. There was nothing I could do about it.

Three weeks later, my white counts were sufficient, and I was back on par with my monthly schedule, but I was scheduled for another Wednesday admission. Guitar wizard Joe Satriani performed in Sacramento five days before my ninth treatment. My friends and I drove down to rendezvous with our friend Aaron Dehart to see the show. Satriani's fingers walked and danced on the guitar fret board like a scurrying spider. The show and the drive away from home were great therapy for my troubled mind.

Some days were better and more eventful than others. I tried to focus on the good and write positive entries to keep my morale up.

4/7/00

Today was a great day; quite long but adventurous. Last night I ate bul-go-gee (a Korean beef dish) and a lot of it. I crashed on the couch before midnight, while watching Jay Leno. At 2 a.m. I woke up and tried to convince myself that I could go back to sleep, but with my crazy sleep patterns, I couldn't. So around 3 a.m., I watched The Sixth Sense, which I recorded weeks earlier.

The movie ended at 5 a.m., but I was still wired as I rewound the tape. As I was flipping through channels, I ran into an infomercial advertising sunglasses. I had been looking for a new pair anyway. A few days ago, as a matter of fact, I was at the mall searching for new shades and was introduced to a pair of Smith sunglasses with three pairs of interchangeable replacement lenses. They were pretty cool, and I figured that $100 would be money well spent on those sunglasses. On the other hand the infomercial presented an even more attractive offer—so good that I just couldn't let it pass by. They were called Mojaves and had six pairs of interchangeable lenses, rather than the three that Smith had. I purchased two sets over the phone for $90, so I could save the extra set for a future gift. I never thought I'd ever buy anything off an infomercial, let alone at the break of dawn. That was the beginning of the day.

I was feeling a little restless. Following the infomercial I e-mailed and looked into fall 2000 admission into UNR and decided what classes I could take for next semester. Next I played my guitar for over an hour. After playing the guitar, I went into the backyard around 8:30 and dug a half-foot of desert hard ground for the water garden. At 10 a.m. I got a call from Jesse and agreed to play nine holes at one o'clock that afternoon. Gene and Brian came along with us. I returned at five in the afternoon and finished digging the remainder of the water garden hole.

I don't know what got into me, but today but I expended energy that I never thought was in me, with so little sleep the night before. It was the most physically active day, besides snowshoeing, since treatment. Perhaps this is a sign saying, "Hey, you'll be better before you know it. It's time to start taking control."

MONTH IX: APRIL 17 – MAY 21
Aquarium

One evening, during spring time Gene Kim and I were watching a TV show called The Naked Chef, hosted by British celebrity chef, Jamie Oliver. He was so widely popular that Prime Minister, Tony Blair, invited him to prepare lunch for the Royal Family. Celebrity chef Emeril Lagasse was very popular around this time as well. While Emeril was famous for saying "BAM", Gene and I noticed that Jamie often said pucker and herbs.

During the spring time I bought a 10 gallon aquarium for the living room. My mom and I picked up four fish at the pet store. One was a plecostomus whom we named Pucker. Another was a lion head gold fish whom we named Herb. The other two were spotted standard gold fish and we named them Salt and Pepper. My mom and I would talk in English accents, which was especially fun when we called Herb, "Hoob", and Pucker, "Pucka".

VENTING A RESTLESS MIND

When the weather consistently stayed warm, I began to dig holes and pull weeds in my backyard. It was very therapeutic, because pulling weeds was like pulling cancer and throwing it in the trash. In exchange I planted flowers, shrubs, and worked on the appeal of our pond by bordering it with slate rock and creating a garden bed.

There were a few days when I made plans to ride my mountain bike in the hills. I had to ride early in the morning because my skin was sensitive to the sun. Speaking of the sun, witnessing the birth of a brand-new spring day is bliss. One privilege of my unofficial sabbatical was the constant availability of spontaneity. Sometimes I'd wake up at three or four in the morning, unable to fall back asleep. Most of the time I read but there were a few instances when I'd walk to a marsh that was over a mile from where I lived to watch the sun rise. It seemed that I was the only one awake in my entire neighborhood. Heck, I was up before the birds. With every passing ten minutes, the sky would illuminate brighter. The dark clouds would transform into oranges and yellows until the sun began to project broad daylight. What a privilege it is to watch the night shadows shrink as the sun peeps its head over the horizon to begin a brand new day.

CHAPTER 15

MUSIC TO MY EARS

I was eight years old when I saw my first live concert. The Beach Boys were my favorite band during my preadolescent years, and I was thrilled when my parents drove us to see them at Caesar's in South Lake Tahoe. I knew the words to most of their songs and sang along. A couple of years later, Pat Benatar performed at the Nevada State Fair while I was with my dad and a friend of mine. I'll never forget the magical feeling when they performed "Shadows of the Night." Without any accompaniment to the vocals, Pat and her assistant guitar player raised one fist into the air and sang valiantly, "We're running with the shadows of the night. So baby, take my hand, you'll be alright. Surrender all your dreams to me tonight. They'll come true in the end." I was mesmerized.

During my freshman year of high school, MC Hammer and his posse of crazy dancers rocked the house at the Lawlor Events Center in Reno. It was my first rap concert and the first time my ears rang for days afterward. I was a huge Hammer fan. To this day I still think his live shows are among the best I've seen, and I'm not afraid to say, "I saw him perform twice."

Live music became my preferred choice of entertainment as I entered my third year of college in 1996. Kyle Archuleta, a friend of mine since middle school, invited some friends and me to see his band, Arch, perform one evening at a bar called the Little Waldorf Saloon, known to locals as "The Wal." Arch began playing the local scene as a punk-metal-alternative cover band. They were extremely high-energy, talented, and a lot of fun to experience live. I was hooked and became a regular.

In 1998 one of my college fraternity brothers, Rodney Teague, was one of the founding members of a local band called Keyser Soze. They had strong ska and reggae influences and brought a different kind of crowd and energy. While Arch made you want to mosh, Keyser Soze made you want to dance, which drew in a lot more ladies.

I rallied my friends whenever Arch or Keyser Soze were scheduled to perform during the school semester. But during the summer or winter breaks, we would drive to Northern California to see the biggest shows come to the West Coast if they didn't pass through Reno. Soundgarden, Pearl Jam, Metallica, Van's Warped Tour, Tool, Social Distortion, Beastie Boys, Bush, Foo Fighters, Rage Against the Machine, Pennywise, Rancid, and Bad Religion were among favorites we saw perform live in college.

In fact when I was diagnosed, Rodney's band made two Keyser Soze t-shirts and gave one to me while I was in the hospital. Kyle also gave me a giant shout out and a huge hug while Arch played at a local club on one evening when I dropped in to say hi. Those were fond moments.

MONTH V: MAY 22 – JUNE 18
One of the Best Shows

Approximately six months before my college graduation and diagnosis, my childhood friend Gene Kim played a CD in his car as we drove home from a ski day at Alpine Meadows. The songs were a very eclectic blend of rap-metal, rock, lounge, ambience, and turntables, and they reminded me of the band Faith No More. On "Redefine," the first song on the Incubus CD, a machine-gun-slapped bass riff engaged my attention. Gene told me the band was called Incubus, and at the time their current album was titled *Science*. I enjoyed Incubus because they had a very appealing sound, they were not trendy, and only a small, esoteric group of people seemed to known of them.

In September of 1999, when I first began chemotherapy, Incubus released a new album entitled *Make Yourself*. In October I went to a Best Buy and purchased three CDs, including the new Incubus album. When I bought the *Science* album a year earlier, I listened to it regularly. When I bought the *Make Yourself* album, I listened to it religiously. It was the perfect theme to my life situation, as the lead singer, Brandon Boyd, sang about the privileges of life, taking control over mental piracy, and being driven. I became addicted and didn't feel my day was complete unless I got my fix. There came a point when I said to myself, "Hey, if I don't stop listening to this CD, I'm going to burn out." I didn't want the inspiration to wear off, so I put the CD back into its rightful case and abstained for a couple days.

In March of 2000 I was browsing the Internet for concerts in Northern California and the Reno-Tahoe area. Incubus was touring with 311 and stopping at the Greek Theater in Berkeley, California, in May. I told myself, "If I could do only one thing this entire year, it would be to go to that concert."

When the month of May began, my white counts were too low, and I was forced to wait an extra week for my immune system to replenish itself. The forced week set me back for a BBBD on May 22. The Incubus/311 concert was May 28, and I contemplated whether I wanted to postpone my treatment for yet another week. If not, I would return from OHSU on Thursday the 25th, leaving me with only two full days of recovery before the show. Regardless, I already bought tickets for my crew and me and hoped I wouldn't experience any serious complications on the way to the show or back.

I came out of my tenth treatment clear-headed and seizure-free on May 25th. The only thing on my mind for the following two days was the anticipation and excitement of the Incubus/311 show. I rested and replenished myself on the short downtime. A total of ten of us were going to the Incubus show. Brandon Barela, Sean O' Hair, Nick Stolpman, Erick Wipf, Jesse Viner, Nick's friend Paul Curry, and I mutually agreed to pitch in and rent a minivan to carpool us for the day of the show. The cost of everything was split evenly between seven of us. My other three friends, Gene Kim, Aaron Dehart, and Ryan Simpson, were leaving later that day to meet us in Berkeley.

Upon arrival we had nearly two hours to spare before the concert began. Sean was familiar with the area and recommended a Thai restaurant, where we visited for dinner. Shortly afterward we strolled among the masses for nearly a half-mile to the Greek Theater. I was filled with enthusiasm, like a little kid on his birthday. The crowd became more congested as we moved closer to the entrance, but the lines moved along smoothly. After walking past an Incubus/311 T-shirt booth, the open-air outdoor venue sprawled out before us. It was like we were in a gladiator coliseum arranged in a semicircle. The flush portion was the stage, which resembled a portico overlooking the fans on the crowded floor.

The show was general admission, and we sat a few seats up and to the side of the sound production booth. Jesse, Sean, Brandon, and I sat one row in front of Nick, Erick, and Paul. It was dusk but still an hour away from nightfall. There was no sign of Gene, Aaron, or Ryan when the lights went out and Incubus stepped on stage. I snuck a handheld tape recorder into the venue and began taping the show when their set began with the song "Privilege." The crowd was into the music, but the movement down on the floor wasn't as animated as I thought it would be. If it weren't for the portacatheter in my chest, I would be down moshing with the crowd. I could barely contain myself. I was in a state of bliss with some of my closest friends, great live music with one of my favorite bands, in the best sounding outdoor venue I have ever experienced for a show.

I knew every word from every song on the *Make Yourself* album and most from the *Science* album as I sang along passionately. Mike Einziger, the guitar player, began a celestial guitar riff I wasn't familiar with, as Brandon Boyd, the lead singer said to the crowd, "You people look absolutely beautiful tonight. This next song is called 'Stellar.'" "When It Comes" came next, before their trademark song "Pardon Me." Boyd didn't wear a shirt for much of the set, and a girl threw her bra on stage at the end of "Pardon Me." Boyd put it on and said, "I don't know, I'm kind of feeling at one with myself right now with this thing."

He continued, "So, 311 is coming up right now," and the crowd became lively. "Let me see your fists in the air for 311," followed by another impressive response. "Let me see your fists in the air for men who wear bras."

Mike Einziger then played an Egyptian-like riff with tribal drumbeats in the background as Boyd sang, "Why am I the only man wearing bra?" I could hear Erick and Nick laughing behind me. Incubus ended their set with "Redefine," the first song I ever heard by the band. As they departed from stage, Boyd commented, "I can't get it off," in reference to the bra.

When Incubus finished their set, I searched for Gene, Aaron, and Ryan for one last time, but we never ran into each other. When the lights went out after setup time, I realized that the fans were mainly at the Greek Theatre to see 311. The volume of the crowd response was enormous when they opened up with the mainstream song, "Down." They were fun to watch, especially with singer/rapper SA Martinez scratching the turntables, singing, rapping, and grooving with every beat. P-Nut, the bass player, danced like a marionette.

311 had been around for nearly ten years before I became interested in their music, but I learned that their fan base is a grassroots following. Other than "Down," the only songs that I was familiar with were "All Mixed Up" and "Beautiful Disaster." Tim Mahoney, the lead guitarist, led an instrumental for warm summer nights called "Cali-Soco," which was very cool and sounded like a Jimmy Buffet song without words.

At one point, Jesse and I walked up to the lawn area to watch the show from higher up.

We sat down and I said, "Dude, check out those lights.

"I know, dude, they're awesome. They look like rotating kaleidoscopes", he replied.

"Like fireflies.

"Yeah."

After performing "All Mixed Up," Nick Hexum, the lead singer, demanded, "I wanna see everyone in this whole place just jumpin' to the beat like one big organism in celebration of the funk." The song was "Applied Science" and began when he said with hype, "Nod your heads to this." There was one part where the drummer, Chad Sexton, tapered off into a solo and the lights were on him only. After ripping it up for a couple of minutes, the lights illuminated the rest of the stage while the rest of the band stood side by side, with their own front of their own drum in front of them, with mallets in hands. Synchronically and progressively, all five band members pounded their drums like an Indian powwow was about to begin. At first the beats came in twos but soon fell into an intense rhythm of twelves and sixteens.

When the song was over, I turned to Jesse and said, "That was pretty dope, dude."

He responded, "Dude, the drums were going right through me." That concert, by far, was the best experience since my time of diagnosis.

Two weeks later Jesse and I drove to Sacramento, where we met Aaron to see Stone Temple Pilots (STP) perform live at the Sacramento Valley Amphitheatre. Papa Roach opened the show. Ever since I was a senior in high school, I wanted to see them in concert. My high school friends and I had several good times at the lake together while listening to STP. I never thought I would get the chance to see them in concert because the lead singer (Scott Weiland) was heavily into heroin, leading to the break up of the band for nearly three years. After some serious rehab, Weiland claimed that his hardcore drug days were over, and Stone Temple Pilots reunited.

STP performed all of their popular songs that evening, and the majority of the crowd sang along to tunes like "Plush," "Sex Type Thing," "Vasoline," "Wicked Garden," "Interstate Love Song," and "Big Empty," to name a few. It was classic!

CHAPTER 16

CONVICTION

MONTH XI: JUNE 19 – JULY 18
Breaking Point

My dad and I flew to Portland on the weekend before my eleventh treatment. We hadn't seen much of Oregon's main attractions, other than the backdrop of Mt. Hood from the hospital. So, on Saturday we toured the Oregon Museum of Science and Industry (OMSI). The museum offered such things as hands-on labs, demonstrations, a planetarium, tropical and deep-sea aquariums, and a tour of the USS *Blueback* submarine, once manned by 85 sailors. Before the day concluded, we saw an Omnimax film, *Cirque de Soleil*, an acrobatic musical performance that depicted life's stages from birth to maturity. We spent the next day at the Oregon Zoo, followed by a walking tour of the intricate Japanese Garden and blooming Rose Garden.

Dr. Kherbache was the neurosurgeon who conducted my Blood-Brain Barrier Disruption procedures since my treatment began. As with all the clinical personnel on the BBBD team, Dr. Kherbache was a very nice, personable fellow, but it was announced in April that he would be gone two months before my treatment was over. He knew of my complications with seizures when either side of my brain was treated, and he was the best at managing them when they occurred; that was important to me. I was saddened to know that he would be gone before my year of chemo was complete. He was always sincere and concerned when asking how each month went.

The month before Dr. Kherbache conducted his last session of chemo on me, I met his replacement, Dr. Kiwic. Dr. Neuwelt introduced him to me while I was in my hospital room, but we exchanged no words, just faithful eye contact. Like Dr. Kherbache, Dr. Kiwic was from Poland. For the first BBBD on the following month, Dr. Kiwic treated the back of my brain, and things went smoothly. The next day was a completely different story when he operated on the side of my brain. I endured three major seizures, the worst sequence yet, with only one month to go.

After I got my first blood test on the following Monday, Cindy called from OHSU to make sure I was taking my Neupogen and Lovenox shots. The phone call was peculiar because no one had called to tell me to continue taking my shots, not since the opening months of my BBBDs. She also asked how my vision was, and I said it was a little hazy, but I knew I had three seizures. I assumed I'd be fine, so I reassured Cindy. Then it dawned on me when I hung up the phone that there was some concern in her voice. I called back immediately to express my concern, and she said my vision should clear up within the next few weeks. My head started playing games with me. I overanalyzed everything that happened and how I was feeling since the previous treatment. Psychologically chemo was wearing me down over the long haul, and I was at a breaking point. I e-mailed my friends to inform them of my inner struggles.

> I'm e-mailing because I've been feeling somewhat depressed since I've been back from Oregon, so I'm venting by way of e-mail. I'm so sick of this chemotherapy bullshit. The good news is that my last treatment will be on July 17.
>
> I don't know. I've been through hell and back too many times this year and I'm really getting fed up with the scene. Can you guys call me or send me something that will keep me positive? I'm starting to feel a little nuts. Anybody interested in going to Warped Tour on Sunday at Boreal? What are you guys doing for the Fourth?
>
> Take Care,
> Danny

I received immediate support and responses from those who had been with me all along. They kept me up. On July 2 I invited Jennifer Enos to come along with me to Boreal to see the Vans Warped Tour. It was her first time and my third. We met up with nearly a dozen other friends and a few other mutual acquaintances. Some of the of the bands we saw perform were NOFX, Green Day, Papa Roach, Long Beach Dub Allstars, Jurassic 5, and the Mighty Mighty Bosstones.

Two days later on the Fourth of July, most of us went to Zephyr Cove in South Lake Tahoe. Zephyr Cove on the Fourth of July is akin to *Spring Break* on MTV: party people everywhere. The weather was absolutely beautiful, as the temperature lingered in the mid-nineties. It had been over a year since I had been to the beach, and I missed it immensely. Around 4 p.m. we ate dinner at a nice restaurant and returned to the beach for fireworks. There were thousands of other spectators along the cool, sandy beach. It was the best Independence Day show I can remember and a fitting celebration to my nearing end of chemo. We drove back to Reno and arrived in town before midnight.

My year of chemo was like a portal for renewal, reflection, and resolve. Besides recovering, what was I to do when my treatment was over? At the time I had thoughts of returning to school for subjects I was interested in, unlike many of the courses I had to take to fulfill a curriculum. The use of my degree in electrical engineering seemed to be a thing of the past because I wasn't very interested anymore. I also wanted to ski that winter and continue to attend concerts of my favorite bands. I needed time to myself to figure out which path I would embark on for the continuation of my life journey. I was a new person with the outlook of an infant who saw the world with innocence. Insight was my head start, but a couple months earlier, I decided that I needed some sort of original belief or creed that I could take with me before I was done with chemo, something to live by. Before I was admitted for my last treatment, I conjured: "What you believe is what you become."

TIME MACHINE

COMING FULL CIRCLE

Before the end of my fourth year as an undergrad, I ran for college of engineering senator and won one of the two available positions. A few weeks after the election, when summer began, I drove to Moab, Utah, with the UNR Outing Club. I wanted to go there ever since high school, when I saw an episode of MTV's *The Real World* ride Slickrock. My friend Spencer Ericksen was president of the outing club, and he organized the trip. There were about a dozen of us, and it was one of the best weeks I ever had. Slickrock was an absolutely amazing ride, with a plethora of mounds of sandstone that seemed out of this world. We rode a 1.7-mile practice ride before we began an approximate ten-mile loop. It was one of the most fun and technical rides I've ridden. It seemed that the ride took me over two hours to complete, and I was exhausted by the time I was finished. Our group rode hard and recovered the next day by hiking around Arches National Park.

The third day we were back on the bikes to ride a route call Porcupine, which was a four-mile uphill followed by a twelve-mile technical downhill. The summit before the long downhill defined the meaning of panorama, as we took moments to admire the vast landscape of towering mesas. It was twelve miles of downhill from there, with four-foot drops along the way. I skimmed over some two-foot drops but none higher than that. Most of the guys in our group were much more experienced than me and had much better bikes. They tore it up.

On the final day we rode nearly 15 miles, but I don't remember the name of the route. It began with a few miles of uphill, followed by a downhill so smooth and fast that I thought I was on a roller coaster. Yes, indeed, Moab kicked ass.

When school began in the fall, I was comfortable with what I had achieved and where I was going, but I was anxious to graduate. *Senioritis had begun.* I enrolled in a yoga class to break the typical monotony of classroom time. School and senate kept me plenty occupied, but I always made time to have fun. I began taking swing dance lessons with a girl named Nicolette Andrini, whom I met the night I won my senate election. Aside from our dance lessons, we practiced at a club that promoted swing dancing. Our routine was solid, and we always raised eyebrows when we danced. Where there was one of us, the other wasn't too far away.

I maintained my 3.0 GPA for the rest of the school year and was thrilled that commencement was near. But we all know what happened before I graduated: Hawaii, finals, headaches, forgetfulness, and shock.

CHAPTER 17

THE FINAL ADMISSION

MONTH XII: JULY 19

Like the previous month, my dad and I flew to Portland two days before admission. We drove to Mount St. Helens in Washington with members of Jonathan's family, Betty, Lionel, and Betsy.

Chemotherapy caused skin sensitivity to the sun and was more susceptible to being burned. On the Fourth of July, I couldn't resist the temptation of taking off my shirt. I rubbed sunscreen on every part of my body except for my chest, which wasn't exposed for much longer than an hour. An hour was all it took to promote a scalding sunburn.

When I awakened the following morning, my chest was beet red and extremely sensitive. I began to regret my carelessness under the sun. A week before I went down to Portland for my last treatment, the burn began to peel, while the area around my portacatheter began to bubble with pus. Accessing my portacatheter for one last time was ugly. My sagging skin was like heated latex, and the range of motion with my left arm before discomfort set in became very limited. Although my port was accessed successfully, the general area looked like scrambled eggs.

I was still concerned about Dr. Kiwic because we hadn't established a line of communication since my seizures from the previous month. I complained to a couple of the nurses on staff and let them know that I was uncomfortable with him. All I wanted was a few moments of social interaction to secure a sense of trust and sincerity. I liked everyone on the BBBD team, and I didn't want to leave chemo with any grudges.

Times were seldom when I felt nauseous during chemo, and the times I did was when I was in the hospital. Nearly halfway through treatment I couldn't bear the taste or smell of food while in the hospital—especially cafeteria food. Chemo patients seem to have a keener sense of smell than most people. It's hard to explain, but there must be some sort of association with the chemicals involved in chemo that make the sense of smell more acute. If I was really hungry, I'd have one of my parents pick up something from downtown Portland for dinner. It was much better than regular hospital food.

Around 9 p.m. on the evening before each BBBD treatment, a nurse would access my portacatheter with an IV line to begin proper hydration before chemo the next day. The IV bag was filled with saline, and my body absorbed nearly three bags each time. At first I could tolerate it, but as the months went on, I'd become more nauseous and sensitive to the taste it left in my mouth. I had a premonition that I would vomit some time before the end of chemo; it was just a matter of time. Water became distasteful. I tolerated apple juice for a couple of months but soon made a switch to cranberry juice. On the last month my options narrowed down to grape juice. Between grape juice and ice water, I must have consumed over a liter that night. I woke up around two in the morning and I hurled purple liquid into a bucket. I felt as bad as it looked. My nurse gave me ice chips to chew on until I fell asleep.

I felt exhausted when I woke up at 7:30 the next morning. Dr. Kiwic, Dr Neuwelt, and a couple other nurses were doing their rounds to talk with each patient before treatment. Dr. Kiwic finally opened up to me and asked how my month went. I told him of my temporary blurred vision from the previous month's seizures. He responded with compassion and was much like Dr. Kherbache. We talked for a few minutes, I don't remember what about, but I felt much more comfortable now that we established a line of trust and communication. I went through chemo with only a mild seizure and felt decent when I came to my senses the next day.

CLOSING REMARKS

In July, shortly after my final round of chemo, my dad sent this letter to family friends and supporters . . .

Danny, Kimberly, and I would like to express our heartfelt thanks for all the support and understanding that everyone has freely expressed and shown in deeds during these last fourteen months.

The treatment cycle for this ordeal is over. It was always difficult and dangerous. We had several frightening encounters which we somehow got through. To wit, as this last treatment had concluded on Wednesday, July 19, early in the morning of Thursday, July 20 Danny came down with a fit of diarrhea and nausea that got everybody's attention. It ain't over till it's over. Fortunately it was dealt with and we were able to catch a plane out of Portland later that afternoon.

The medical community is very upbeat because there is no detectable evidence of disease. Most importantly, various flavors of CT scan and MRIs have been clear and unchanged for six months. During August 15-17 we will return to OHSU, Oregon Health Sciences University, for a beginning to end clinical review of Danny's case. In attendance will be the key members of the BBBD staff, Blood Brain Barrier Disruption. Additionally there will be more tests and appointments with an Opthamologist, Danny has slight double vision on the vertical, and a Neuro Physiologist, to measure brain functionality. On both counts Danny is in pretty good shape with time and therapy expected help even more. It wouldn't surprise me if there was a little party in there too.

Currently, Danny is completing for the last time the monthly post treatment regime of medications, steroids, and self injections. The steroids are the worst, can't sleep, rashes, uncharacteristic mood swings, and exaggerated appetite. In a week or so these too will be never more.

The remainder of 2000 will be a period of recuperation and reflection. He just submitted an initial proposal to Readers Digest in an attempt to eventually publish his Regarding Hope essay. No easy task because it is a very competitive step by step process. There is on-going contact with other patients, most still undergoing treatment, and volunteer work with The Leukemia and Lymphoma Society. In late August he will begin taking a few classes and seminars at the University and perhaps a part time job.

Beyond the year 2000 is wide open and full or opportunity. With what he has been through Danny is forever transformed but in most other ways he is still the same ol dude. Aunt Rose Marie, the Nurse Practitioner who really runs the BBBD program day to day and is somebody we deeply respect and love, said things often happen for reasons we don't immediately understand. We'll take that.

-Ted

CHAPTER 18

EASING BACK INTO LIFE

FOLLOW UP

Needless to say, the end of chemo was a relief, but it was business as usual for the next month: Neupogen and Lovenox shots, six-hour doses of Leucovorin and Decadron, daily doses of Dilantin, weekly blood tests, inconsistent sleeping patterns, mood swings. My hair would fall out for one last time.

Ten days following my last treatment, several friends and I would drive to the Sacramento Valley Amphitheatre for a Dave Matthews concert on July 30. The trip was planned months earlier and I looked forward to it as much as I did the Incubus and 311 show in Berkeley that previous May.

Our tickets were general admission, which put us on the lawn in the back. Luckily others from our party arrived earlier that evening to secure a vast area with blankets. It was a very ceremonious and joyful time for me. Twelve months of chemo had finally past as I was now breathing the air of freedom.

Three weeks later my parents and I flew to Portland again. It was one last official follow-up that included an MRI, a chest X-ray, another ophthalmology appointment, and a quick meeting with Dr. Neuwelt. "I don't want to see you here again," he said, with somewhat of a smirk. It was all for good intentions that I had rid my brain of cancer. I returned to ward 5A for one last time to say hi and bye to all the nurses. As usual they were all very kind and happy to see me.

I also met with Dr. Guastadisegni, a.k.a. "Dr. Paul," for a closing evaluation of my cognitive functioning. It was the same test he had given me a year earlier when I first began chemo. The difference was like night and day, as all of my scores improved immensely from my baseline evaluation.

Processing complex information and performing multitasks climbed to average from extremely low and below average. According to Dr. Paul, my improvements were substantial, and it was reported that I would most likely make a thorough cognitive recovery.

BACK TO SCHOOL

Jesse and I enrolled in a music-recording class at UNR that semester. We wanted to play in a band at some point in our lives and thought that such education was right up our alley. It was my partial way of keeping busy and diverting my mind from stagnation. There were over a dozen students in the class, which was twice as many for the fire safety code of the recording studio. Because the interest was more than anticipated, the instructor decided to add another section. I was among one of the first to sign up and permitted in the first section without question. Jesse was not, so I changed sections so we could work on projects together.

Recording music is an endeavor as much as it is an art form, and it's much easier to learn with an effective teacher. Our instructor liked to hear himself talk more than he liked to teach. He was very knowledgeable, but his lectures were hard to follow. Sometimes when someone asked a question, he would reply condescendingly, "I told you a hundred times. Don't you take notes?" Taking effective notes from his lectures was like assembling a jigsaw puzzle without a picture to look at. When it was time to put them together, we were left with questions to topics that our instructor claimed he covered. He was extremely vague when it came to making a point.

On the bright side I learned to record music and apply techniques with assignments. Through the class, however, I discovered a deficiency in my cognitive redevelopment. I had difficulty processing, comprehending, and responding to technical audible information, and I often leaned on Jesse to get me through. I became frustrated and insecure with my ability to learn. This music recording class was the first true test of how my cancer ordeal effected my competency before diagnosis.

CAUSE AND EFFECT

In the ocean when the tide is receding, waves pull in rather than push out. As time rolled by, the process of my mental recovery resembled a similar analogy. Often I found myself in a riptide of anxiety. Any psychological development, lack thereof, or chemical imbalance that affected me after chemo actually began during chemo. Sleep deprivation, lack of social interaction, living in the future rather than the present, thoughts of my inevitable expiration of health insurance, loneliness, aspirations of travel, poignant emotional reactions from Decadron, anxiety for my portacatheter to be removed so I could play sports again—it was all a vicious cycle. Repeating patterns replayed themselves day in and day out. I was quite overwhelmed.

It is said that for every day a patient goes through chemo, it takes just as long to recover. In my case it was a year. My whole psychological outlook during the first year of remission kept me close to the shelter of those taking care of me: doctors, nurses, family, and friends. I was closer than ever to my mom, who was and always has been the most nurturing person in my life. She spoiled me with love, kindness, and freshly cooked meals. My dad was unconditionally by my side to support me in any endeavor. Outside of family I didn't ask for much materialistically. I was too proud to ask for help and didn't want to burden others with my emotional struggles. I suppose in a lot of people's eyes, I was an inspiration but who would be qualified to give someone like me guidance to move forward with my life? At that time there were no resources for young adult cancer survivors to turn to. There was nothing, not even within the American Cancer Society and the Leukemia & Lymphoma Society. It seemed anyone who had cancer was either a child or folks in there 50s or older.

Post-mandatory procedures were important, and I was obligated and steadfast to them as I eased back into a normal life. After chemo my head was never in the past; it was in the future, and that caused a lot of anxiety. I wanted to be there now. Week after week Europe would be lingering in my thoughts. I was stubborn, and it weighed heavily on my resolve to live in the present. The more I thought about it, the more depressed I became. Nearly a year had passed until reality set in with more negotiable expectations. There was a lot more going on than physical recovery and wanting to go to Europe. I wasn't happy, I wasn't sad, but I often felt isolated and unsure of how to carry on with my life.

Psychologically war seems to have the same ramifications, whether it's through mortar and gunfire or battling through cancer. When the war is over, psychological and emotional scars can run deep. I was in a state of post-traumatic stress disorder. I began to understand what it was like when soldiers returned from war and how difficult it could be to get back into the swing of life.

Returning to normal, consistent sleeping patterns and mediating to a normal state of chemical balance were chores I longed for. Physically and mentally, normalcy was a concept that I was unfamiliar with for quite some time. Imagine living day to day with only two to four hours of sleep per night for an entire year. Then imagine a drug that stimulates random mood swings within that time. When you want to sleep, you can't because of all the reckless energy caused by the Decadron. It caused a lot of anxiety and sometimes made me over-analytical. Subconscious scars of that kind don't heal overnight; hence I'm sure you can see why I became frustrated in my music-recording class. Such a disorder wrought havoc on my cognitive retention as I tried to return to a regular life. But my life would never be regular again after all I'd been through. How could it, and why would I want it to be?

During my five years of college, I was constantly busy, with little time to sweat the small stuff. I was socially interacting with people every day, and I thrived on it. When I was diagnosed with a brain tumor, the attitude I conveyed to others was a positive one, and no one ever questioned my tenacity to get through chemo. Without them, I'm not sure if I would have made it sanely. As my months of chemo progressed, my social network was reduced to a few friends whom I talked to or hung out with a couple times a month. But they, too, had their lives to get on with, while I was waiting to start mine after riding an unimaginable roller coaster of emotions, medical drama, and trauma.

For a short while after chemo, my sleeping patterns improved to uninterrupted nights of eight to nine hours. A month had barely passed from my last admission on July 17, and I was enrolled in two classes at the university: music recording and yoga. I was completely tapered from my doses of Decadron but prescribed with hydrocortisone, a milder steroid that also reduced inflammation and swelling. It would be nearly a year before I was permitted to abandon all medications except for Dilantin. In fact, I would have to live the rest of my life with a seizure-risk condition.

Class time at the university comprised three hours of my week. Aside from studying, that left a lot of time to think about things, perhaps too much time. I had no job, no girlfriend, and no immediate goals. The only thing I resolved myself to thinking about was writing my book, traveling to Europe, getting my portacatheter removed, and the possibility of returning to school for advanced education. Lack of action based on the convictions in my mind was my worst enemy. I was left with a lot of time to think, and quite frankly it's hard for me to remember where the time went or what I did with it.

The analogy I conjured in my head was a slingshot. While I recovered, I'd have to walk backwards to prepare for my new life, and when I was ready, I would let go and launch into my vision. I envisioned myself being a writer for an adventure or concert magazine. I also envisioned myself as being a motivational speaker to share my story of overcoming cancer and moving on. But those visions became blurred through anxiety and depression.

The year following my last round of chemo was as difficult as the year of going through treatment but on a different psychological scale.

Although I survived the trials of cancer and chemotherapy, it was difficult finding a community to bond with. I struggled through more than a year of melancholy and diminished self-esteem. But I remained hopeful and continued searching for a vessel to carry me through.

DROP THE LEASH

Under doctor's orders the portacatheter in my chest would remain for a minimum of three months post-treatment. I wanted it out ASAP, so I could get back into physical activities that chemotherapy constricted me from. Basketball, tennis, skiing, softball, and volleyball were sports I looked forward to, but the portacatheter in my chest was a liability. I couldn't risk a hard hit that could knock it into a lung. I had much anticipation and no patience to get it removed. I wanted to tear it out.

October 25th was a day of conservative elation. The plastic implant that had been lodged inside my chest for thirteen months was finally discarded. Dr. McElreath, the man who implanted the portacatheter in my chest, had just returned from family business in Oklahoma. He worked a half day, and I was one of the patients he dealt with upon his return. Four o'clock was my appointment time, and my mom and I arrived fifteen minutes early to fill out paperwork. It wasn't all that bad, just a page to verify insurance and emergency contact and demographic information. A rare occurrence took place when I was called to the back before my official appointment time: the nurse directed me down the hall where Dr. McElreath would perform the procedure, and rather than go back with me, my mom decided to remain in the waiting room.

The nurse and I made small talk as she prepared all the instruments necessary for the procedure. She asked me the inevitable question: "Why do you have that? Chemotherapy?"

I replied bluntly, "Yes." It was unavoidable, so I went on, "Yeah, I am in my third month of remission." I gave her the one-minute disclaimer that I gave to everyone else: three craniotomies, one year of chemotherapy at OHSU, glad it's over. I went on to tell her that my treatment didn't involve radiation, just chemo.

"How do you feel?" she asked.

"I feel great. I'm just easing back into it."

She replied how her nephew had been in a situation similar to mine.

When he was eighteen and a freshman in college, he had a brain stem operation that involved radiation, but I didn't bother to ask about any details. Instead she told me he was doing great for about seven years but slowly started to lose it. That was unwelcome information I didn't need to hear. I felt blessed that I didn't need to go through radiation.

By 4:30 my mom entered the room because the nurse informed her that Dr. McElreath was running behind. She decided to keep me company, and five minutes later the doc arrived with his assistant.

"Should I stay?" my mom asked.

"You can stay, go to the waiting room, or whatever," McElreath replied. I asked my Mom to leave, and she said, "That's good. I don't want to watch, anyway."

Dr. McElreath applied cold alcohol to disinfect the skin around my left chest muscle. He draped a 3 x 3-inch dressing window to isolate the targeted area and grabbed a syringe with a two-inch needle and asked if I was ready. "Yes."

"Little poke," he followed.

Little poke my ass. I squeezed my fists and looked away to divert the pain as Dr. McElreath pierced my flesh and immersed the syringe an inch into my chest, at a slanted angle. He swiveled the needle like a lever and injected lidocaine while casually talking to his assistant about the weather and the fish he caught down in Oklahoma. After pulling the syringe out of my chest, he punctured me two more times. This lasted for about thirty seconds as I squirmed with pain and adrenaline. Afterwards I glanced down at my chest. It was somewhat swollen like a breast without a nipple. A minute later, Dr. McElreath said that my chest area should be numb by now. *It better be.* "You shouldn't feel a thing. If you do, let me know and we'll take care of it, but you shouldn't feel a thing. You shouldn't feel a thing, except for a little tugging and pulling," he declared.

I could've looked down to watch but chose not to, as I felt the scalpel when it glided through my skin. Next, I felt the picking and pulling of my flesh. Although my chest was numb, I could feel the catheter slither out just above my heart. Now that it was out, I asked if I could take a look before it was thrown into the biohazard wastebasket. It was a white plastic ring with the circumference of a quarter, a centimeter thick, and attached to its catheter like a Life Saver candy on a rope. It was my lifesaver from being a human pincushion during my chemo treatments.

Dr. McElreath sealed the incision with what appeared to be a miniature welder. The scent of the fumes took me back to my adolescent years at the dentist office when a cavity was being drilled. It reeked like drilled tooth. Next he sewed me up with a suture that would dissolve within the next two weeks. After removing the dressing, he cleaned the affected area with alcohol and layered a clear plastic adhesive. For the next 48 hours I wasn't supposed get it wet; therefore no shower for two days. The only discomfort I experienced was a mild bruising sensation that night. I was excited and thankful for its removal.

HIGHLIGHTS FOR THE REMAINDER OF THE YEAR

Skiing was one thing I absolutely wanted to get back into when winter came around. The Mt. Rose ski resort offered a killer deal on a season pass for only $200. Plus the drive from my house was only twenty minutes. It was an offer few people in town could refuse. I waited in line for over two hours the weekend they went on sale, reading *National Geographic Adventure* magazine as the line slowly crept forward. Along with my bald, bloated, and scarred chemo head, I stuck my tongue out when my picture was taken for the ski pass.

Although it wasn't as frequent, my concert going lifestyle remained as an anchor for optimism. Days before the fall semester began, Gene, Aaron, and I drove to San Francisco to see Zebrahead at Slims. For the remainder of the year, I saw Third Eye Blind, Live, the Counting Crows, Bad Religion, Incubus, the Deftones, and Pearl Jam with my usual group of friends. Then on December 2, I saw Tina Turner with my mom and dad.

From the time I began chemotherapy in August 1999 until the end of 2000, I attended 14 concerts. The cost of my rock n' roll lifestyle during that time totaled approximately five hundred dollars, but it was money well spent. It was music where I was happiest as I marched down the road of cancer.

PRELUDE TO GREATNESS

A couple of times during my eleventh and twelfth months of chemo, I went to the gym to try indoor cycling classes on a stationary bike. These indoor cycling classes was part of a fitness craze called *spinning* where endurance workouts are accompanied or choreographed to music. The sign on the door to the spinning room quoted, "Burn 500 to 800 calories in forty-five minutes." Spinning classes simulate road rides with varying resistances, resembling steep hills, bumps, and downhill terrains. At the time they were new to me, and they were a good way to break the monotony in a day. The 45-minute classes were extremely challenging and tiring, but I felt renewed and baptized with sweat at the end of each class.

The first two classes I attended were in the late afternoon on Sundays during chemo. A month after my last BBBD, I began attending noon classes regularly. They were held on Monday, Wednesday, and Friday, and I typically went on two of those days. The instructor was Kim Nance, and she had a big following. Nearly two dozen bikes would be used for each class. Sometimes late arrivers would be SOL. Kim was an amazing energetic "soccer mom" type with a family, and she treated everyone as a friend. She asked for names of new, unknown faces so she could address them more personally. Everyone liked her, and she inspired the thought of becoming a spinning instructor myself.

A MOMENT TO REFLECT
Life Lessons from a Brian Cancer Diagnosis, Three Craniotomies, and a Year of Chemo

There are many milestones in life. A brain cancer diagnosis after college graduation contained many milestones in itself. Learning to talk and write again, realizing I could read again, retraining my brain to play the guitar and piano, writing an essay, surviving three craniotomies and a year of chemo all epitomized my grandest of milestones during this time. But they also taught me many timeless lessons:

- You must have hope.
- Being there can make all the difference in the world.
- It's OK to cry.
- Life is right now at this very moment. It must be embraced to experience.
- Friendship is an ideal that delivers courage and advances new levels of motivation, thinking, and feeling.
- What you believe is what you become.
- To grow you must learn to become comfortable with being uncomfortable.
- Embrace change.
- You must take the path least traveled to find out what you're made of.

PART TWO

The Years: 2001 - 2010

CHAPTER 19

LETTING GO AND MOVING ON

THE SEARCH FOR SALVATION

Jeff Dawson married in January 2001, and I was his best man. Since second grade we have shared many life milestones, such as learning how to properly "flip the bird," getting kicked out of class, basketball camps, high school graduation, and seeing him off when he joined the air force. Now I had the privilege to attend one of his biggest milestones: his wedding.

After our first semester in college, Jeff joined the air force for the opportunity to see the world. I remained in Reno for a college education. Since 1995 he has been stationed in Biloxi, Mississippi, Texas, the Carolinas, Saudi Arabia, Bosnia, Germany, several other countries, and the U.K., where he met his wife-to-be, Rebecca. Jeff was the first of my closest friends to get hitched, and of course I wanted to be there. But I was still living off social security disability benefits, so a round trip with accommodations was far from what I could afford. I told Jeff's mom, Sharon, that I'd love to go, but financially I was insecure. She insisted that I go and offered an all-expenses-paid trip. "I want you to go," she demanded.

If Jeff were to have it his way, there would have been three best men: Chris Crawforth, who I was supposed to backpack Europe with; another close friend named Todd Michaelson, who was now a certified PGA golf instructor; and myself. Chris couldn't make it because he recently started working as a full-time ranger in Phoenix, Arizona. Although in town during the Christmas break, Chris was unable to stay for the wedding. Duty called. Todd didn't realize the urgency until Jeff came to Reno for the holidays. He, too, had work obligations. Then there was me, in remission.

Jeff's family and I stayed at the Stanley Hotel in Estes Park, Colorado. It was founded by Freelan Oscar Stanley, the entrepreneur who invented the Stanley Steamer automobile. It was a good history lesson, but I was more familiar with the hotel as the inspiration for Steven King's horror book *The Shining*. In a way I was in a similar mental state to that of Jack Nicholson's movie character. I was the recovering chemo patient, and Jack was the recovering alcoholic. I was also becoming stir-crazy after chemo in my own house.

Each room at the Stanley had its own unique layout. Jeff and I shared a room, except for the night of the wedding. Sharon's room was occupied by Jeff's dad, Lou, and grandma, Mona. Jeff's sister Shannon, her husband Don, and their ten-month-old daughter "Sammy" shared one big room with a breakfast table and a bathroom big enough to be another bedroom.

As Jeff and I grew up, I remember Shannon as an outgoing party girl who was always coming home late, sometimes sneaking in through her bedroom window. Jeff and Shannon are six years apart in age with Shannon being older, a big enough difference to be considered almost a generation gap. I found it humorous that, no matter what, Shannon and Don would name their child Sammy regardless of gender, like Sammy Hagar from Van Halen. Shannon was also a big AC/DC fan. She told me on the weekend of the wedding, "Even if you don't like AC/DC, you should see them perform live . . . if they ever play again. It's incredible."

The wedding and reception took place on the outskirts of Estes Park, 72 miles northwest of Denver, at the Inn of Glenhaven, within the vicinity of the Colorado Rockies. Like the Stanley, the Inn of Glenhaven was built in the early 1900s, and both were favorites for weddings. I felt very fortunate and truly grateful for the privilege to be there for one of Jeff's biggest life milestones; his wedding.

CHECKUP – JANUARY 15

The twentieth of January 2001 would be the six-month anniversary of my cancer-free remission. However, it was hardly anything to celebrate until I knew for sure. Before my departure for Jeff's wedding, I made prior arrangements to see Dr. Conrath upon my return. Since my last treatment he wanted to closely monitor my recovery and overall state of being. For standard yet mandatory medical protocol, I was on a hydrocortisone taper and continued with regular doses of Dilantin. I was anxious to abandon all medications, but Rose Marie at OHSU once said, "Dilantin would be the last medication you'd stop taking."

Days before my appointment with Dr. Conrath, I went to the lab for blood work. At my visit he said, "Everything looks good, except your Dilantin level is at 0.9." My adequate range was between a 10 and 20. It was 90 percent less what it should be. "You're flirting with danger," he stated. "You could lose your driving privileges, especially if you were to have a seizure on the road." I couldn't argue. Despite my own personal ego, I had to listen to the doc. With Jeff's wedding and all I became lazy and careless about my meds. Dilantin never made me feel different or anything less—I was just stubborn. In addition my white blood count was adequate but not optimum to support a sufficient immune system.

Rose Marie mentioned, "For every month you undergo chemotherapy, it takes just as long to recover." Six months down, six months to go. I also had a rash on my right temple, which had been there for about a month. Conrath tentatively diagnosed it as either a rash or strange fungal infection. He prescribed a medication called Ketoconazole cream. If the blotch didn't go away within the next couple weeks, he would refer me to a dermatologist. But it did go away . . . weeks later.

SOBER LUMBAR PUNCTURE – JANUARY 16

The day after my follow-up with Dr. Conrath, I felt conflicted: I dreaded it but looked forward to getting it over with. Six months of remission had passed, which meant it was time for an initial follow-up spinal tap. Every time I thought of it, I couldn't help but reflect back to what happened in

UCLA, when a resident punctured a nerve in my lower spinal column.

The initial spinal tap of remission was scheduled for two in the afternoon on January 16, 2001. At first I planned to drive myself to the hospital, but a nurse at Dr. Conrath's told me over the phone, "You need to have a ride."

"What do you mean? Can't I drive myself?" I replied in frustration.

"You nee . . . "

"OK, fine," I replied in irritation. I was told to check in a half-hour early. My mom was off from work that day, so she would be my escort. She wouldn't have approved of me going alone, anyway.

The lumbar puncture I was about to undergo was much different than any of the previous ones. Rather than roll onto one side and curl into the tightest ball possible, I was instructed to lie flat on my stomach with a pillow under my belly. I asked about the different method and the technician replied, "This is called fluoroscopy. It allows us to greatly enhance the accuracy of the procedure." Instead of going in blind, fluoroscopy involves a real-time X-ray that allows a doctor to accurately control and see where the needle is being placed. I mentioned my experiences with my other lumbar punctures, and the tech seemed surprised to hear that they were performed blind. He did agree, however, there was always a chance of hitting a nerve or artery, but fluoroscopy greatly reduces that risk. Dr. Noh would carry out my procedure, and according to the tech, I was in good hands.

It was the hurry-up-and-wait game, as it usually was with most of my doctor appointments, and I tried to relax until Dr. Noh arrived. Meanwhile, the technician said it was necessary to shave the little amount of hair on my lower back for a clean operation. Nearly a half-hour after the scheduled time, Dr. Noh finally arrived. Although he was late, we had a common trait and interest, which settled some of my anxiety. He was Korean, and we both had degrees in electrical engineering. After earning his bachelor's at the University of California, Berkeley, he continued and completed medical school at John Hopkins in Baltimore. I was convinced I was in good hands.

The technician sat on the other side of a glass window while communicating with Dr. Noh through a microphone. I was shifted up, down, left, and right until my back was aligned in the proper crosshairs. The procedure began when Dr. Noh disinfected my lower back with Q-tips soaked in Betadine, a cold sensation. Immediately following this, he said, "OK, Daniel, a little poke and some stinging." Shallow injections of numbing medicine burned and stung my lower back as I tried to breathe steadily.

Thirty seconds later, Dr. Noh proceeded, "You should only feel pressure, but if you feel pain, let me know and I'll numb you up more." He began to penetrate the big needle through the intermediate layers of my spinal column. When it was at the proper depth, I was instructed to bear down, as if making a bowel movement, so spinal fluid would secrete from my back. After a few tries, Dr. Noh withdrew the needle as I breathed a sigh of relief, only to find out that nothing seeped. That gave me some grief, especially when I was told that he had to go up to the next vertebra and try again. Once again the needle was immersed into my back as I bore down some more. After a few long minutes, spinal fluid finally filled four tiny bottles. He commented how hard it was to penetrate the needle into my back, harder than most, but that meant I had strong bones. He also mentioned, "Usually my patients are a lot older, so it's much easier to draw fluid."

After the procedure I was sent to a recovery room on a gurney. It was mentioned that the last thing I should do after a spinal tap is walk around, unless I wanted a roaring headache. Meanwhile I nodded off and on, as I waited for nearly three hours with my mom by my side, until I was permitted to leave the hospital. That was the easiest spinal tap yet. After six months of remission, I was cancer-free.

BABY STEPS

Recovery was hard. When chemo was over, I allowed myself an entire year before launching a job hunt for meaningful work. Although my mind had shifted from my ambition to backpack Europe, I was still anxious to accomplish something different and convincing. My thoughts wandered with no certain direction or confidence. I enrolled in a swimming class at UNR to train for a triathlon. I also received a CPR/first aid certificate in April because I aspired to train to be a river guide for the summer. That would be my compensation since I let go of Europe. Perhaps after the upcoming summer I would come full circle.

It was nearly February, and the only thing I had on my weekly agenda was a swimming-for-fitness class, skiing with Jesse and/or Gene, and occasionally exercising at the gym. I had a learning curve to overcome in my swimming class because I never learned the proper technique of freestyle. My friend Liz Welsh from student senate was in the class, and we trained together in the remedial section of the pool. The instructor had a close eye on everyone and was quick to point out errors in technique. I had to learn how to breath properly while maintaining proper mechanics. By the end of the semester, I had a more solid technique, but I was still among the slowest.

There needed to be more sustenance in my everyday life. I began looking for work and community service after my 25th birthday in February. The only thing good about turning twenty five was the reduction of my car insurance. One day when I was walking around the university, I saw a flyer on a bulletin board seeking volunteers to encourage kids to read. The program was called Read & Succeed, and I was delighted for the opportunity to give my time. After consulting with an administrator of the program, I was given a choice of schools to work for, so I chose the one closest to the university. That way I could go there without having to worry about being late for my swim class. My duty would be to meet with a few elementary school-children separately one day in the week. I would spend twenty minutes with each child, taking turns reading to each other.

A month before I accepted the gig for Read & Succeed, I began looking for work, hoping to find something related to my degree in electrical engineering. I wasn't ready for a full-time job, just something to help the time pass. One day when I returned from the gym, my neighbor Pete was in his front yard, and he asked what I was doing. "Not much, just coming back from the gym and looking for a job." Pete told me of a private engineering firm that he was doing contract work with for the school district and invited me to go down there to check it out. The company was called Jensen Engineering, and Pete said he would call the owner and mention that I was interested in an interview. Like most of my days at that time, not much was planned, so I was spontaneous in my actions. Immediately after talking to Pete, I showered, shaved, dressed appropriately, ate, printed my resume, and drove to Jensen Engineering, which was only a mile from my house.

I would work for the firm for about three months as a draftsman to catch up on backlog. During this time it became clearly evident that life as an engineer would not make me happy. Draft work was boring and tedious.

I began the Read & Succeed program and Jensen Engineering on Wednesday, March 7. The night before, Gene and I drove to Caesar's Palace in South Lake Tahoe to see a band called Ozomatli. We drove back to town the same night. The next morning I met with Doug, a parent of one of the kids in Read & Succeed. He was a nice guy who was a pleasure to talk with. The first day was to get to know the kids, so he gave me the names of my students and a "Getting to Know You" form for the first day. It was a good icebreaker that asked about favorites (movie, color, book, etc.), age, nickname, activities, and ideas. My kids for the semester were Hailee, who was a six-year-old first-grader, and David and Gary, who were both eight-year-old second-graders.

My experience working with kids wasn't much at that point, but Read & Succeed was a great learning experience. Each of the kids were very different, and each week presented a different challenge to keep them interested. Hailee was shy, David loved to talk, and Gary was very attentive. There was a big box of books, and I let them choose which ones they wanted to read or vice versa. Reading aloud to me was their primary obligation, while I encouraged and helped them with words they had trouble pronouncing.

After the first couple of weeks, I learned that I needed to make each of my meetings different. It was so easy for them to lose their interest or become distracted. When their attention strayed, we played tic-tac-toe or connect the dots before we read. When *that* began to disinterest them, I learned a couple of magic tricks. Making a ball disappear from a vase, transforming a penny into a dime, a couple of card tricks, and reading their minds brought wonder and motivation. I performed a different trick every week. Puzzles and interactive reading workbooks kept them interested, too.

After the first two weeks, I could tell that Hailee was becoming more comfortable and motivated to read with me. Eventually she began to greet me with a smile. The program wasn't much of a problem for David. Gary would give me a hug after most of our sessions. Read & Succeed was rewarding because it added sustenance to my life, and I was able to contribute my time to the community.

SEIZURE

I played softball in a very competitive league in college for a team that was made up of a lot of my fraternity brothers. They invited me back to play in the spring of 2001. During the middle of the game, a pop fly was hit in my general direction and was easily playable for an out.

But as the ball rose up into the lights I began to have a mild seizure that escalated into a dizzying ordeal. The ball landed about five feet away from me, and I tried reaching for the ball about five times but I couldn't grab it. I lost nearly all of my depth perception. By the time I grabbed the ball, the lead runner was nearly at second base, and I tried to throw the ball to the cut off man. The next thing I knew, I was on the ground spinning as if I stepped off of a state fair ride. I didn't get up as my teammates rushed to the field. I couldn't speak because of the seizure. Many of them were there for me when I was first diagnosed, and it was decided to call for an ambulance. Halfway to the hospital, I began to regain my senses and ability to speak.

My parents picked me up from the hospital and I was back to normal after a couple days.

SELF-EVALUATION

The world I lived in before college graduation was compatible with the aspirations of my future. Electrical engineering positions couldn't be filled fast enough along with average starting salaries in the mid $50,000's. Along with great starting pay and corporate employee benefits it seemed my future was bright with stability.

But after cancer, chemotherapy, and recovery time, the world was much different. For one I was no longer a fresh college grad, and by the time I went out looking for jobs, they weren't as easy to come by. I had nearly two years without work experience. The dot.com bubble had burst, and the market was saturated with technical specialists. Most entry-level jobs were claimed by those who possessed advanced degrees and/or had prior related work experience. My two year old bachelor degree in electrical engineering was practically obsolete in the new job landscape.

Something else that added to my frustration was my aspiration to go to Europe. I had to face the fact that the time for me to go came and went.

I made the decision to see a therapist, but after my second session I realized what she was telling me was something I didn't already know. It was a waste of time, and I couldn't afford $110 per session. I would have to figure things out on my own. So, instead of making life more complicated, I taught myself the art of letting go to simplify my state of mind. My aspirations to backpack Europe weighed heavily on me, and I still hadn't felt a sense of closure since I finished chemo. That was my time to celebrate a life milestone but that time had come and gone. Life wasn't waiting for anyone as people moved away, went to grad school, travelled the world, or were beginning their careers.

As an only child my mom and dad had been through enough, taking care of me during my time through diagnosis and chemo. I kept my feelings to myself because the last thing my parents needed to hear was, "I'm not happy." My mom would have trouble sleeping any time I ever told her something was wrong, and I simply did not want to burden her. Whatever decision I chose to make would be supported by friends and family.

I wanted to experience Europe with friends, but now there was nobody to share it with, at least at that point in my life. I was doubting and second-guessing myself to move forward because of it. Europe was holding me back and I realized it was time to let go. The liberation from that decision was monumental and it was a huge stride in my recovery. I learned that the art of letting go is an art, indeed.

LIFE WITH TEAM IN TRAINING

New possibilities began to unfold when I relieved my mind of traveling to Europe. Nearly two months following the marathon in Sacramento, early February 2001, I was invited to another kickoff party for *Team in Training* (TNT), still as an honored patient. I talked Liz Welsh into coming with me because I knew she was into endurance events and the whole fitness thing. We were former college senators who served in the same term the year before we graduated. By coincidence we enrolled in the same swimming-for-fitness class, which was where I first mentioned and began to talk about TNT.

Team in Training had a new area coordinator by the name of Kelly Anderson. She was extremely genuine and motivated to make sure everything ran smoothly, and she did an excellent job.

The training season kickoff party offered sandwiches, drinks, and various other finger foods to tie the event together. Before presenting the honored patients, a video was shown to inform and inspire those who would train for the first time. The vibe and intention of *Team in Training* video was very positive and personal to me. On the video people of all ages glimmered with smiles and motivation as they ran or cycled and then finished a marathon or a century bike ride. It left me choked up inside. I barely fought off tears but shed one or two by the video's end, hoping no one would notice, and pretended to rub my eye. Living through cancer the way I did empowered me to give back—maybe not at the moment but someday. After the video the honored patients were asked to stand one at a time to be recognized and be applauded by the fifty-some-odd attendees. It wasn't until the end of the official announcements that I was able to meet other members of TNT.

There were two younger women running in my honor. One named Rachel was quick to ask questions for what she could do to learn about or help me. Shalee, who was more reserved, went to high school with me when she was a freshman and I was a senior. I met both of them for the first time. There was another girl whom I knew because she played softball for our high school; her name was Brandy. Aside from that, I learned that TNT also had a coach for a cycling team by the name of Dan Brown. I shared some of my riding experiences and skill level, and mentioned that I had ridden Moab.

Dan owned a local bike shop called Bicycle Bananas where TNT members were entitled to a store discount, which I thought was pretty cool. Despite the fact that I had been exercising moderately, I was in no state of mind to train for a twenty-six-mile marathon or a century bike ride. However, I was running frequently for my own personal good. Five miles was the distance I was comfortable with at the time.

A month after the TNT kickoff party, I decided to run with the pack one morning. They ran every Wednesday evening and Saturday morning. The team was at fourteen miles on Saturday mornings, but I was welcome to join at any time for whatever distance I felt I could handle. When the run began, I took off at my normal pace, beginning at the tail end of the pack. Before I knew it, I was running alone and passing most. I began to feel left out at approximately three miles, so I stopped and waited for Shalee and Brandy. I felt that maybe I could run 10 miles that day. I had no idea what I was getting myself into.

At approximately the halfway point, Shalee turned back to prepare for her brother's wedding; otherwise, she said, she would have run the entire fourteen. There were five or six of us when Shalee and a few others turned back. Brandy was planning to run the entire fourteen miles for that day. I was feeling pretty good at seven miles, so I decided to run the rest with

Brandy—or so I thought. Never before in my whole life had I run that far, and I was about to find out whether or not it was a good idea.

One additional mile passed and some others turned back, then I felt the tendons behind my knee joints begin to tighten. Brandy took a short breather with me as I guzzled some water and massaged my own legs. We proceeded a couple more miles into a residential neighborhood, and my legs tightened up even more. Eventually I began to walk as Brandy went ahead, but she ran bonus miles to check up on me.

I was dying with about three miles to go, and my joints felt like they were grinding. To be honest, I was miserable. When I finally lugged myself to the starting point, I thanked Brandy for helping me get through the long run, and we went about doing our separate things for the rest of the day. I knew I was due for a few days of recovery, but I didn't think I would come out as sore as I did the next day. That night wasn't too bad, although my legs were feeling on the heavy side. I was so broken down the following morning that it hurt to walk. I felt nauseated and completely exhausted. Nearly a week passed before I began to feel like myself again. Running wasn't something I enjoyed any more.

ORDINARY TO EXTRAORDINARY

Cancer illuminated realizations and spontaneity. It's impossible to ignore the fact that our lives travel through time and windows of opportunity. To me it's vital to realize opportunities and take advantage of their benefits, but timing is everything. While undergoing chemo, Gene Kim and I philosophized about how spontaneity was the spice of life. Spontaneity is the will and curiosity that adds a dynamic to life. Spontaneity is a key that can unlock doors leading to a greater vision.

Since the year began, I had attended Jeff's wedding, worked part-time at Jensen Engineering, swam for fitness, donated my time to Read & Succeed, and not much else (except a Linkin Park concert). I felt edgy and not yet over the aftereffects of chemotherapy. During the middle of May I decided to take a week off from work and head south to attend a couple of concerts in Las Vegas and Los Angeles. It was the first time I would break away from home on my own since remission.

Brandon Barela was planning his exit strategy from Reno and move to Las Vegas, so he rode along with me on the way down. He would stay at his stepbrother's house and fly back to Reno days later. Meanwhile I spent time with my Aunt Sherre and cousins Windy and Michael. Windy and I saw David Gray and Nelly Furtado at the Joint inside the Hard Rock Casino.

The following day I departed for Southern California, where I would stay at my Aunt Joan's house in Westlake, hang out in Santa Monica spending time with Aunt Melva, and see Dave Matthews perform at Dodgers Stadium. I stayed at my cousin Don's house for a night in the Bay Area and drove back home to Reno the following day. But when I returned home, I didn't feel like I accomplished much, and I was back to feeling somewhat depressed.

My south-and-back road trip ended a day earlier than planned, which was a Thursday. That was a good thing because I had a three-day weekend to recoup before I would have to return to work on Monday. The Leukemia & Lymphoma Society was gearing up for the big weekend that they had trained for since the beginning of the year: the marathon in San Diego and the century bike ride around Lake Tahoe. Another TNT kickoff party was held on the following Wednesday, the last one for the month of May. As an honored patient, I was encouraged to attend once again.

The get-together was in a conference room at Washoe Medical Center. There, I met up with all those whom I met after the beginning of the year at the season kickoff party. Shalee, Rachel, Brandy, Kelly and Dan were all there along with the rest of the team, supporters, and other honored patients. I also met the coach of the running group, Ski Pisarski.

I'd say there were forty people who showed up. Two other guys by the names of Ed and Greg trained for the century bike ride, and I met them for the first time. That evening Dan Brown invited me to visit his shop some time before the weekend. "We'll help you pick out a bike and you can ride with us around Tahoe", he offered.

The last time I had ridden a road bike was when I was in middle school, and that was around the block. It wasn't even my bike. Dan said, "You're more than welcome to ride with the team; as far as you want [on the day of the ride]." I graciously accepted with no high expectations. At most my intentions were to ride 25 or 30 miles. I certainly didn't want to put the same physical strain on my body like I had on that 14-mile run.

The next day I went to Dan's shop and was fitted on a brand-new, blue-and-white Fuji road bike. On Friday I rode about ten miles around my neighborhood, so I could get a feel. I couldn't believe how much power I had, despite the bike's lighter weight in comparison to a mountain bike. The spinning classes I attended after chemotherapy truly revolutionized my riding, and I have Kim Nance to thank for the inspiration. Plugging in the technique and power that was required to tread through Kim's indoor classes made the real road feel like air. I was definitely riding at an entirely new level.

The century ride is an annual one called "America's Most Beautiful Bike Ride," and it was scheduled to begin at 6 a.m. on Sunday, June 3, at the Horizon Casino in South Lake Tahoe. Ed and Greg raised the appropriate funds during their training period and had an all-expense-paid weekend: hotel, pasta party, breakfast, ride support, and after-party. They didn't hesitate to let me crash in their hotel room on the night before the big day.

Dan and I rendezvoused at the Horizon on the night of the pasta party. We arrived late and walked into the ballroom during the middle of the presentation for *Team in Training*. From the looks of things it appeared that nearly a thousand people attended, and Dan and I found the rest of the team towards the back. I treated myself to a generous serving of salad, pasta, and dessert. Meanwhile a few speakers addressed the crowd with information, such as road rules, safety, tradition, and top fundraisers. I ate until the last speaker came to the podium to talk about his child who had leukemia. I don't remember the details of his speech, but I could feel the anguish that my parents went through as he began to weep. It was very emotional and I even shed a couple of tears. The man received a well-deserved standing ovation.

I didn't sleep too well that night because I was in an odd place on the floor of Ed and Greg's hotel room. The next thing I knew, the alarm was buzzing at 5 a.m., and the sky was still dark. Ed and Gregg didn't seem to have a problem with rolling out of bed, but I sure felt sluggish. I crawled out of my sleeping bag half an hour later. In the lobby of our hotel, bagels, fruit, and OJ were served for *Team in Training* participants. Without a *Team in Training* jersey like everyone else, I was condescendingly looked upon as a poacher. I grabbed a bagel, cream cheese, banana, and a small carton of OJ when one guy sarcastically mentioned, "Sure, why don't you go ahead and help yourself? You deserve it." There were six or seven people looking at me like a criminal. I replied, "I'm an honored brain cancer survivor," pointed out the scar on my head, and walked away.

The tour around the lake began at 6 a.m., as groups of riders launched in waves according to geographic origin, every five minutes. Riders from Reno were part of the greater Sacramento area chapter, and we were the fourth wave to go. Ed and Gregg were strong riders, and there was no way I could keep up with them. Dan was an experienced rider, too, but he opted to stay back with me. As we began the opening stretch, he asked what my story was, and I told him. Obviously Dan knew I was an honored patient, but I had a full head of hair and seemed normal like anyone else. In exchange for my testimony, Dan told me his own life story. We established a genuine bond.

The weather from the past few days was fairly nice, reaching highs in the mid-70s to low 80s. A 2000-foot altitude gain from Reno to Lake Tahoe enhanced the briskness of the morning. I wore the fingerless mountain bike gloves and helmet from my mountain biking days in college. My body was dressed in layers, beginning with a T-shirt under two long sleeves, covered by a windbreaker. My legs were layered with shorts, sweats, and nylon parachute pants. I also brought along the Camelback I wore during my college bike rides. All in all I was enjoying myself riding among two thousand others.

For nearly ten miles the road was flat, until a slight grade pulled up for nearly two miles. The next two and a half miles was a four-hundred-foot elevation gain full of switchbacks. I was passing the vast majority of the riders along the zigs and zags, and I lost myself in my own ego. I lost Dan, too. Emerald Bay loomed between the passing trees, the sun was rising, and it was impossible to ignore the splendid scenery. It was the most beautiful spectacle I had seen since remission. The next mile was a fast descent leading to the first rest stop at 14 miles, Inspiration Point. I took a leak, hydrated, ate some orange slices, a half-bagel, and a banana. Hundreds of others were doing the same, but I couldn't find Dan. I really didn't know what I was in for or what the day would bring me.

If I were to turn back and return from the way I came, I would have ridden a total of 28 miles. Others would be continuing the journey around the lake, while I was at the hotel taking a nap. Then I would wait for hours until I found the rest of the team in the afternoon. That would be a worst-case scenario. But there was a default within me that urged me to keep going. If need be, shuttles were available all day, and I had that option if I couldn't go on. Turning back meant failure to me. I certainly wasn't trained to ride 100 miles, but nothing could be lost in an attempt. Physically I felt terrific, but I had to find Dan to keep me going. I couldn't stay motivated going alone. After waiting for nearly ten minutes, I spotted Dan at the rest stop and signed in relief.

We proceeded to ride, and he offered a couple of riding pointers. Drafting is a technique that team riders use to conserve energy during long rides. One rider leads to break the draft from the followers. After certain distances the riders switch roles, while one leads and the others follow. In our case it was just the two of us, as we practiced for a short while along the way. He also noted to get into the habit of pointing out debris along the road, especially when leading the pack. Grates and covered manholes were everywhere.

We reached the second rest stop at 25 miles, the Homewood Mountain

Resort, where I shed a couple of clothing layers. Empty plastic bags were available for participants who wanted to leave clothing items behind. I ditched my windbreaker, a long sleeve, and my two layers of pants, leaving me with shorts and a short sleeve under a long sleeve. We refueled for a short while and proceeded.

Dan told me that, after the next half dozen miles, the road split off in two directions. One detoured to Truckee and added the difference to complete the full 100-mile tour. The other continued along the perimeter of the lake, which would total a sum of 72 miles. At that point I was over 31 miles into the ride. If I rode back the way I came, I would have ridden over 62 miles. If I continued for another five miles, I would be halfway around the lake, and there was really no point in turning back. My mileage would equal the same either way. The lunch stop at Kings Beach was 11 miles away, so I figured to at least make it there and figure out the rest as I went along. I was beginning to feel weary, and a meal would do me some good. Dan was awesome, as he decided to continue riding with me rather than ride the full century. I was grateful. Besides, he had plans to ride a century with his girlfriend the following week on a tandem bike.

Within an hour we were at Kings Beach, and I was starving. Hundreds of riders were mingling and eating. Sub sandwiches, water, energy drinks, brownies, and fruit were readily available to participants. I ate a foot's worth of sandwich, a brownie, and drank loads of water. A nap seemed like a good idea. Dan informed me that we had nearly 30 miles to go after breaking for over an hour.

After riding a few miles, I felt the onset of fatigue, then I tried GU. GU was one of the sponsors of "Americas Most Beautiful Bike Ride," and that's exactly what it is, *goo*. It comes in disposable packets of various flavors, and it squeezes out like gel. I had the vanilla bean flavor, which was surprisingly good. Before a minute had passed, my body had metabolized it, and I felt rejuvenated as if I awakened from a power nap. The GU was power packed with a 100-calorie, 25-gram carbohydrate. It was my second wind.

Ahead of us was a 12-mile climb with an elevation gain of 700 feet to Spooner Junction. Because I had been to Lake Tahoe more times than I can remember, I was well aware of the ascending stretch. It was a whale of a hill, and I had to give it all I had. Dan trailed as I began the climb with the applied mentality of the spinning classes I participated in with Kim Nance—maintain cadence. Dan commented, "You're looking strong." There was a water stop three miles into the climb, but I refused and pressed on. My legs grinded away as I took sips from my Camelback; I felt possessed and had no desire to stop until I was at the top of the hill.

My body was well beyond its riding capacity, and I was really starting to feel it. The contrast between passing the world from a car window compared to being in a bike saddle was very distinct. It took longer to travel from point A to point B, but details of the open road were more relevant from a bike. Every stretch of climbing was like carrying a bag of rocks that got heavier with each mile. Mentally I was at one with myself, listening and feeling every part of my worn-down, aching body. My legs felt like lead and my joints like rusted hinges. Just when I thought I would reach the summit, another ascent would be a football field away. But I was the little engine that could. *I think I can, I think I can, I think I can.*

The ride up Spooner that day was the hardest 12 miles I have ever ridden. It was a chore, and I yearned to alleviate the heaviness of my body and legs. I was immensely relieved when I finally spotted the masses of riders and cheering fans. The rest stop was the last of the ride, and nearly ten miles remained. Incoming riders were greeted by cheering supporters. I ate a small Balance Bar, drank a lot of water, and lay on the warm pavement. My body nearly melted into the parking lot, and I wanted to sleep forever. Dan and I were there for nearly 20 minutes, until I finally peeled myself from the ground.

By the laws of gravity, what goes up must come down. I knew that most of the remaining trek was home-free, beginning with a few miles of pure downhill and a loss of 700 feet in elevation. Well, not exactly. When driving down it, I always shifted my truck into a lower gear, so I could coast and minimize the use of my brakes. I always wondered what it would be like to ride down Highway 50 on a bike, and now I finally had the chance. The wind blew hard against us that day, so it was difficult to gain speed. My concentration was fully focused on my line while steering clear of grates. I simply held on for the free ride. I'm sure I reached a speed I never had prior to that descent. A few minutes later we approached a landmark known as Cave Rock. Two gaping holes are blasted into a mountain to create a tunnel to allow traffic continuity around the lake. I howled as I passed through. From there the big hill began to peter out into a gradual two-mile ascent. In fact there were several rolling hills before us. Psychologically this was somewhat frustrating.

Soon we stooped into another downhill that led to Zephyr Cove Resort, the same area I received my sunburn before my final month of chemo. The traffic light at the bottom of the intersection was red; my legs felt more oxidized than ever, and they screamed for rest. I'm sure Dan read my fatigue by my facial expressions and body language. He asked if I wanted to take a break, but I refused and continued when the light turned to green. I was over my limits as we continued onto another ascent. A few minutes later I couldn't take any more, and I had to stop for a short while. My legs felt like papier-mâché that had been beaten like a piñata.

We pulled to the side of the road as I got off my bike and lay on my back. I apologized to Dan and said, "Sorry, my body just isn't trained to ride this far."

"Don't worry," he answered, "This is for you. We can rest for as long as you want." Dan had no doubt in his mind because we were only two to three miles away from the finish line. But for me, whatever distance remained seemed to be an eternity. At that time I just wanted to get the ride over with. We were about three miles away from South Tahoe.

Nearly fifteen minutes later, I crawled back onto my bike through exhaustion beyond belief, and we continued. From past driving experiences, I always know that South Shore, Lake Tahoe, is near whenever I saw the two tennis courts off to the side of the road. That's when my mentality shifted to autopilot. We weren't much farther, and I couldn't believe that I was about to complete the 72 miles ride around Lake Tahoe in a single day. Initially I felt a tremendous sense of relief but the final stretch around the last bend opened up to a meadow that was my gateway to rapture. I could finally see the casinos of South Lake Tahoe where the ride began.

Dan trailed as I pedaled faster; I wanted to finish strong. The bend slowly began to straighten into a 300 yard home stretch that ran through the gut of downtown. The time was about 3:00 p.m., as supporters and families of riders cheered and applauded like we were soldiers coming home from war. I sure felt like one and howled my loudest, *Wooohoooooo!* and raised my fists into the air. Nobody knew me, although hundreds of onlookers rooted and cheered with enthusiasm. Like a crescendo, a tsunami of emotion began crashed into me. Tears began to stream down my face, and it was the best feeling of my entire life.

Before I allowed myself to get off my bike, I had to embrace Dan. I couldn't thank him enough for what he helped me achieve. He was like a saint. Ed and Greg finished the 100-mile tour in a respectable time, and they, too, were there to greet us.

Through spontaneity the day was perfect. A few steps away from our little congregation, masseuses stood by for sore riders, but there was a short line. I waited fifteen minutes, then relished one of the best leg rubdowns I ever had. For the same amount of time, my quads, calves, hamstrings, and feet were worked over by well-trained hands. It hurt so good to have the knots rubbed out, as I chuckled in pain. My legs felt light as a feather when I began to walk again, and that was only the beginning of my indulgence in luxury. I was encouraged to hang around for the after-party. How could I refuse? "Next year, you've got to do the whole thing," Ed said.

Before I could engage in any more fun, I needed to get in a little R&R. Ed gave me the key to the hotel room so I could take a nap. Our room was on the tenth floor or so. When I peered out the window, I couldn't believe it; the room overlooked an executive wading pool and three Jacuzzis. Did I die and go to heaven? I slept heavily for nearly an hour and awakened feeling like a blob of lethargy, yet filled with excitement. I couldn't miss the opportunity to sunbathe, indulge in a Jacuzzi, and spoil myself in the buffet of pasta, steamed vegetables, salad, and desserts. My body seemed to metabolize food at the very touch of my fingertips. And the Jacuzzi, well, that was celestial. I was in ultimate self-pamper mode.

Ed and Gregg's families were laying around the side of the pool, relaxing and savoring the moment as well. Dan came and went. I was happy to be in their company. The entire day was a welcoming atmosphere, and it didn't end at the pool party. There was more to come, beginning at 6:30 p.m. with a victory celebration. I went back to the hotel room, slept for another hour, showered, and headed down to the ballroom, where TNT participants would celebrate the day.

It was a bash. All of us were on the dance floor at one point or another. Dan danced more than any of us, as if he was on the prowl. Ed and Gregg were scheduled to work early the following morning. They departed from the party at a decent hour and left me the key to the hotel room. The following morning I called into work and reported that I was coming in late.

SETTING PRIORITIES

Finishing America's Most Beautiful Bike Ride was the most significant moment of my life. According to the release of his book at the beginning of 2000, Lance Armstrong made a statement to the media when he finished his first tour: "If you ever get a second chance in life, you've got to go all the way." I took that to heart when I rode the 72 miles around the lake in 2001, and I carried it with me into 2002.

My version of going all the way would be to train for the entire 100 miles the following year through *Team in Training* and raise money for the allocated fundraising goal to benefit the Leukemia & Lymphoma Society.

A few days later, I reconnected with Jeff Cooney, Curtis Fuestch, and

Jonathan Yasui to let them know my plans for the 2002 ride. I planned to ride in their honor. It was then I learned that Jeff's body rejected his stem cell transplant, and he had an awfully tough time recovering. Finally it got to a point where his chemo treatment was doing more harm than good.

Jeff informed me that the doctors gave him two choices. One was to continue treatment; but the cancer was so advanced and his body so broken down by chemo that his immune system might not recover. Or he could discontinue chemo, stop the suffering, and live the last few months of his life in peace.

I was saddened in September when I heard of his passing and it made my decision to raise money for the Leukemia & Lymphoma Society much more meaningful. I would dedicate my ride to his memory.

I enrolled in a full course load that fall semester to help advance the development of my cognitive abilities and possibly embark on a career path in teaching. I enrolled in a history class, expository writing, music vocal class, and military science 101. The contrast of university life between my college graduation and returning to start all over again was culture shock for me.

Prior to diagnosis I spent five years at the university. I had a routine, social skills, and a large network of friends in the college community. By the time I finished chemo and attempted to go back, all of that was diluted. I didn't know anyone on campus any more. All of my friends had graduated and were getting started with their careers. The student body when I returned were mainly of freshman and sophomore age, and I had a difficult time accepting that I was now 25 and everyone else was 18 or 19 years old.

What I knew for sure was my mission with *Team in Training*, and thanks to the inspiration of Kim Nance, I would become a certified spinning instructor in December 2001. I immediately made the sub list for two local fitness clubs at the beginning of 2002.

CHAPTER 20

2002 - A NEW FOUNDATION

From honored patient to active participant, I became instrumental to recruiting efforts with my story for *Team in Training*. Our cycling team was 12-strong by the end of January, and each of us were obligated to fundraise a minimum of $2,200 in order to participate in the event. Participants were bound by a fundraising contract that stated if an individual didn't raise the minimum amount, they would need to find a way to pay the difference. People from all over the United States trained and raised money to ride around beautiful Lake Tahoe.

Coach Ann Conlin was from New York and was an Ironman finisher, which at the time was an inconceivable thought, yet very inspiring. Ann had our group on a regimented weekly training agenda leading up to our century bike ride on the first weekend of June. The midweek rides were difficult to bring everyone together because each person had their own set of family and work obligations. But on the weekends most people were free, and we'd make a progression in mileage every weekend. We began with 15 miles then worked our way up on a weekly basis.

I personally felt the fitness progression each week. If we jumped from a 40-mile ride to a 50-mile ride, I'd have to push hard to finish the last five miles. But the next time I rode 50 miles, it wasn't as much of a chore. My longest training ride of the year was 85 miles two weeks before the century.

Team in Training gave me my first genuine sense of community since my final treatment in July of 2000. It was the only constant in my life, and I felt like part of a new family. The team gave me confidence and a solid sense of purpose, and I finally felt like I was making a turn for the better. Nothing much really mattered except to finish what I set out to do. The only thing I knew for certain was I needed to finish that ride in memory of Jeff Cooney, in honor of Jonathan Yasui and Curtis Fuetsch, and to bring a sense of closure for myself. I figured if I kept a healthy and active lifestyle, my chances of long term survival would be optimal.

At approximately 8:30 on Thursday evening, April 11, the phone rang as I was checking my e-mail. It was Betty Walkit's voice on the other end. Immediately I knew why she called because at this point no news was good news. Jonathan had passed away at 8:30 that morning, and Valerie wanted us to know. The news was the extent of the entire conversation. I walked into the living room to tell my dad. He was lost for words as much as I was. I walked into my parents' room, where my mom was removing her make up. She, too, was startled. After we received Betty's last e-mail four weeks earlier, my mom intended to call and see how Jonathon was doing; but she never got to it, although it was always in the back of her mind.

My dad tried to return Betty's call, but the line was busy. He called Valerie instead. I don't know what she said on the other end, but it shook up my dad and brought him to tears. I had never seen him so shook up to a point where he couldn't hold back tears, as he handed the phone to my mom. I gave him a hug as my mom finished the phone call. We all hugged and held a few moments of silence. My father thought it would be appropriate for me to attend Jonathan's funeral in Portland, Oregon.

I initially had intentions to make plans, fly up, and attend the funeral. Initially we were under the impression that the funeral would be on the following Tuesday. The day following the news, we received an e-mail from Valerie that the funeral was scheduled for the upcoming Monday.

Months earlier, I made plans to drive up to Sacramento and see my favorite band, Incubus, in concert with two of my good friends. My father said, "Well, you better change plans." Because I never expressed my melancholy or internal feelings to my parents, they didn't understand my reasoning. But my mom's instincts and premonitions knew I was still in a vulnerable and fragile state of mind.

I was angry and saddened that cancer had taken two of my friends within a year. At that particular time in my life, attending the funeral to miss the concert would leave me with regret and resentment. Call me selfish but I wasn't going to let cancer ruin more of my plans. I was only 26 years old, less than two years into remission, and damn it, I still needed closure.

Jonathon and I had a special bond, and I would understand his decision if the circumstances were flip-flopped. We understood more than anyone that our days were numbered and to enjoy life while we could. I decided not to go to the funeral and instead to enjoy an opportunity to be happy at the Incubus concert with two of my closest friends.

Jonathan and Valerie were like extensions of immediate family. After a day of contemplation my parents decided to make plans and drive up to Portland rather than fly. My mom would be off from work by 5:30 on Sunday afternoon. Dad would be home during the course of the day in preparation for the drive to Portland and back.

In total the twelve members of our team raised over $30,000. I raised over $2,700 by the time of America's Most Beautiful Bike Ride, which was $500 over my fundraising goal. Once the fund-raising minimum was reached, each participant would have an all-expenses-paid trip for travel, accommodations, and food related to the event. The 2,000 people who came to Tahoe raised over $8 million for the Leukemia & Lymphoma Society, just as the group before them had in 2001.

Team in Training held a pasta feed for all of the participants at the various host hotels in South Tahoe on the evening before the bike ride. There were guest speakers to get the crowds excited and to reflect upon the reason why everyone trained for hundreds of miles. They spoke about the course, safety, and appreciating the moment. They also had an honorary speaker whose life had been affected by cancer. In 2002 I was chosen to speak the evening before the race. My mom, dad, and Uncle Don would be there to celebrate the occasion.

I shared my story about headaches, diagnosis, craniotomies, and chemo. I also shared my experience of riding around the lake in 2001 and how much it meant to finish. When my story reached the tennis courts in South Tahoe, I fought to hold back tears as I described the casinos that would soon come into sight near the finish line. Before I could finish the speech, I paused to re-gather myself when all of a sudden, the crowd of 800 rose in a standing ovation. There wasn't a dry eye in the room.

I concluded my speech with Lance Armstrong's quote when he finished his first tour, "So, this year I'm going all the way. I raised the money, I put in the miles, and tomorrow I'm going to ride 100 miles. See you on the road."

I received a second standing ovation as I stepped down from the podium, shaking hands and high-fiving those along the way. I hugged my mom, dad, Uncle Don, and my teammates upon my return to our table.

Team in Training athlete participants would be issued a registration bag upon arrival at packet pick-up. In the packet would be an assigned bib number, helmet stickers to match the bib number, an event water bottle, event long sleeve shirt, and advertising collateral from presenting sponsors. Most TNT participants also wore an honorary bracelet for the patient they had been raising money for. I wore four: one for Jonathan Yasui, one for Jeff Cooney, one for a young child named Sebastien Garcia who was battling leukemia, and one for my fellow survivor, Curtis Fuetsch.

In honor of Jonathan's memory, Valerie sent me a picture of him on a fishing boat in Hawaii. He was smiling and flashing the hang-loose hand sign. I wore that picture on my Camelback throughout the entire ride in his honor.

During the event I would also be somewhat of a celebrity around Tahoe because of my speech. I received several accolades throughout the day along the 100-mile course and even in the elevator and buffet lines after the ride.

My personal mission to finish that 100 mile bike ride and to increase awareness through my battle with cancer gave me a full sense of closure. From that point forward, life began to open up with opportunities I could have never imagined.

A CAREER OPPORTUNITY OF A LIFETIME

Kathryn Bricker oversaw the group exercise activity of several clubs in the greater Reno area, and she hired me as a sub once I became a certified spinning instructor. I met Kathryn through a mutual friend who also instructed spinning. She knew that I eventually wanted to earn my own weekly time slot and was willing to pay it forward to prove that I was worthwhile. Tuesday and Thursday evenings at 5:30 p.m. were my ideal times.

Toward the end of December 2001, I was contacted by an old high school friend who needed a sub for a 6 a.m. class at Nevada Fitness on Wednesday, January 2. It was an early morning after New Year's, but I gladly accepted.

There were about six people who attended my first class. I was a little nervous and reserved at first. I had a few issues getting the stereo to work properly, but I was able to resolve them and get the class started about five minutes later than scheduled. In the end it didn't matter because everybody expressed their appreciation of good music and high intensity.

The very first song on my repertoire was "Thunderstruck," the live version by AC/DC. I needed to begin the class with a bang after starting late. I played ten songs that went on for the duration of nearly 45 minutes followed by a ten-minute cool-down stretch session.

A couple of weeks later I was contacted by another instructor who requested I sub for her Monday morning class at 6 a.m. Upon completion of the class, one of the students by the name of Seth Sheck complimented me and said, "Dude, you play kick-ass music. You should take over this class. I love the energy."

"Thank you," I replied and blatantly admitted, "One of the main reasons I wanted to instruct was so I could play my own music. I'm glad you enjoyed the class."

I was humbled and excited by Seth's compliment. He reaffirmed my passion for wanting to instruct spinning because I was able to exercise, motivate people, and, best of all, play my own music. I accepted every opportunity to sub for other instructors' because I knew that it was only a matter of time before a permanent class would become available. Every so often Seth would attend my spinning class, not necessarily because of me but because it was part of his routine of staying in shape. He was always very enthusiastic when I subbed.

After I rode AMBBR at the beginning of June, it had been well over a month since I was called to sub a class. Then at the beginning of August, I was contacted to sub another early morning Wednesday class. Seth was there again. After class, Seth and I continued to chat as we walked out into the parking lot, and he asked me, "So what do you do?"

I didn't have much to speak for at the time, but I mentioned, "I'm working at Lowe's part time in the garden department. It's a retainer job to give me flexibility as I trained to ride my first century bike ride."

"What do you want to do?," Seth asked.

I validated myself, "Well, even though I have a degree in electrical engineering, my dream job would be to be a writer for *Rolling Stone* or *National Geographic*."

"Well, I work with *Pollstar Magazine*, PLSN, and I have connections in the music industry." That struck a chord with me because I was already familiar with Pollstar. Pollstar is an online concert search engine. If a band is on tour, it will display all the dates and locations where it's performing. I used it frequently while in college.

He went on, "What kind of music or bands do you like?"

"Incubus, 311, Creed."

"Dude, those are my clients," he exclaimed.

So, at this point I was interested, yet cautious. I had been down a similar road in college with a friend of a friend who was big into network marketing. I invested about $1,000 in student loans, which I never saw again. Lesson learned because, if it sounds too good to be true, it probably is. "Well, what do you do?" I asked.

"I own a company that designs and manufactures security credentials and backstage passes, called Access Pass & Design. We opened our doors for business at the beginning of the year." It did sound too good to be true, especially in Reno, Nevada. *Backstage passes out of Reno? Really?*

He was completely transparent and explained his predicament, "I generate the majority of sales in the company, but my sales cycle is a constant grind of peaks and valleys. I'll ramp enough sales to keep my department afloat, but I also do all the admin work, which includes writing up a quote, sending it to the client, closing the deal, micromanaging it through the shop, inspecting it, and billing it after it ships. It's a grind, and I need someone who can manage all the admin work for me so I can focus on new sales and developing relationships. The micromanaging just kills my time. I need someone to help." I was catching his drift, and I was optimistically cautious about the potential of this opportunity.

Part of me thought, "I've survived brain cancer and chemo, and the last thing I'd ever want to do is become someone's assistant and documents papers." Yet another part of me thought, "This has potential and who knows what doors this may open in the future?"

"I'm definitely interested," I said to Seth. He gave me his card and invited me to swing by the shop. "Come on down. I'd be happy to show you around." I went home, showered, ate breakfast, printed out my resume, and showed up less than two hours later, wearing slacks and a polo shirt.

Access Pass & Design was located in one of the several suites in the Oakcrest business complex. Upon entering the office suite, there was a vacant desk in the front. To the left was an office occupied by a sales exec. Seth came out from the back to greet me and began showing me around the facility and introducing me to his partners and coworkers. There were framed sets of passes of various clients that Access Pass & Design was working for, including Incubus, 311, Creed, Pink, Laguna Seca Mazda Raceway, *American Idol*, and a few British properties, such as the Scorpions, S Club 7, and *Pop Idol*. All this was proof that Seth was the real deal, although it was all somewhat surreal at the time. It reminded me of what it might be like to enter an office at MTV. It was exciting!

I called Seth the next day to accept the position, with the understanding that I needed to give Lowe's my two weeks' notice. My first official day at Access Pass & Design was on Monday, August 12, and I didn't work any more than ten hours per week until I finished my final two weeks at Lowe's. At the end of that first week at Access Pass & Design, I had a free ticket to see Chris Isaac at the Reno Hilton Amphitheatre, courtesy of the company, and I hung with Seth and some of the other Access employees at the show. Not a bad way to start.

I got busy living in 2002 and never looked back. And as a result this book was put on hold for many years. Essentially, my life was just about to begin through an adventurous career with a start-up company and a progressive lifestyle through endurance sports.

CHAPTER 21

AN UNLIKELY CAREER

LIFE WITH ACCESS

The story of Access Pass & Design is an inspirational one of a small business, perseverance, partnerships, perks and luck. Seth Sheck, Brad Diller, and Frank Himler started the business because they knew they could do it better than where they came from. Led by Seth, the company's persistence created luck and when the opportunities were ripe, the owners were swift to capitalize on them. That included acquisitions, finding professional consultants who knew how to build businesses, and good old fashioned hard work.

Access Pass & Design had its fair share of growing pains over the years but the three owners always found a way to rally and find resolve at varying degrees of sacrifice. Interestingly enough, they compensated for each other's weaknesses. Where one needed improvement, another excelled. This was important for company balance.

Seth was a pistol who moved the company forward. He was the eternal optimist and wouldn't take no for an answer.

Brad had the loudest personality. He was vocal about speaking anything on his mind, yet was a creative and swift problem solver.

Frank was the most technical and analytical of the three. I often sought him out when I needed clarity with any process.

I became Seth's right hand man during my first five years with the company. We'd often travel to San Diego, Long Beach, Las Vegas, and Los Angeles to establish a greater presence in the concert touring business. Seth taught me that the best business at those conferences happened at the bar. That was the best area for networking because you never knew who you would meet. In the conference environment, days would often begin at 8am and end at midnight to 3am the next day depending on what was happening. It was grueling at times but always interesting.

It's tough to beat a job that pays you to watch concerts, hang out backstage with rock stars and groupie chicks, and watch artists perform while actually standing on stage during a performance. From 2003 through 2006, I had backstage and onstage experiences with the Black Eyed Peas, Jack Johnson, Ben Harper, Slightly Stoopid, Pennywise, Bad Religion, KISS, Foo Fighters, Godsmack, Fiona Apple, Incubus, 311, G. Love, The Roots, Eek-A-Mouse, John Butler Trio, and Queen. I became the guy that my friends lived vicariously through. But one of my all time favorites was in 2006 when Seth and I were in Vegas one year and we were comped floor tickets to see The Rolling Stones at the MGM Grand; 9th row back, center aisle.

Over the next three years business travel allowed me to experience several U.S. cities for the first time, including Philadelphia, Houston, Nashville, Phoenix, Ft. Lauderdale, Austin, and Atlanta. I would also visit New York City and Aspen twice each within those three years. Although I had prior visits to Las Vegas, Seattle, Los Angeles, Long Beach, and San Diego, business travel would bring me back to those cities as well. I particularly enjoyed this part of my job which enabled me to network on a national level, and learn about other U.S. cities. In fact, business travel through Access was filling the void I lost with Europe because of my cancer diagnosis.

The music industry was Seth's passion. I loved music and sports so I had the best of both worlds, but the company hardly had any sports clients. Over the next three years I would find myself working in both industries. Seth granted me free reign to build our business in the sports market. And as time went on, I would become more withdrawn from the music industry to take on a business development role in sports.

By the end of my second year at Access in 2004 I had won a third of the college bowl game market including business from The Rose Bowl, Gator Bowl, and GMAC Bowl. But the key to my success in breaking into the sports industry came through partnerships in the sports conference space.

Seth found his way to success in the music business the same way and he fully supported my endeavors to make a name for Access Pass & Design in the sports industry.

During the summer of 2003 Frank, Seth, and their spouses went to New Orleans for a conference called IAAM (International Association of Arena Managers). They met with a facilities manager for the Superdome, home of the New Orleans Saints and the Bayou Classic. The Bayou Classic was an annual college football game that took place on Saturday during the Thanksgiving weekend between the Grambling Tigers and the Southern Jaguars. The Superdome and the Bayou Classic became clients that I managed soon after that trip.

IAAM came to Reno in 2004, and Seth brokered a partnership deal: badges for a booth. Because the event was local, Access Pass & Design benefited greatly with a larger presence of employees. The return on investment was three times more than what we put in.

During the conference an energetic woman named Lisa Furfine approached our booth and asked if I'd be interested in being a part of her conference in a capacity similar to that we had with IAAM. "We love your badges, and they would be a great upgrade to our event." She explained that the conference she ran was called TEAMS (Travel Events and Management in Sports). "If you like the type of attendees at IAAM, and if you're looking to get into the sports business, then you need to be at our event."

I was ecstatic and told her that we were looking for new partners to help us get into the sports industry. Lisa handed me an information packet to present to the owners. Little did I know at the time, the encounter would later prove to be the biggest break of my career.

After bringing the opportunity to the owners and corresponding with Lisa on a partnership decision deadline, I got the green light to proceed and make it my own. Just like Seth had been partners with several conferences in the music industry, I put the company's first partnership deal together in the sports industry. I was very proud of that.

TEAMS took take place in Houston during the third week of October. I learned a lot more about the market that TEAMS catered to as I got comfortable networking at the event. The conference attendees were convention and visitors' bureaus (CVBs), sports commissions, hotels, transportation companies, national governing bodies (NGBs), and event organizers. In short, TEAMS was a hub where all of those entities gathered to showcase their cities, venues, and hospitality accommodations so that they may host events such as the Super Bowl, X-Games, and Olympic qualifiers.

I would proceed to network in the usual fashion, and I shared with the folks I met that Access Pass & Design was responsible for providing the badges. Many were impressed and requested more information.

TEAMS is an extremely social event, with plenty of opportunities to network outside of tradeshow hours. One of the social events took place in Toyota Center, home of the Houston Rockets. Attendees had free reign to tour the facility, enjoy an open bar, buffet and hors d'oeuvres. They also opened up the basketball court for attendees to shoot hoops, which was especially cool. The World Series also took place during that time, so after the networking session in Toyota Center, all the attendees gathered downtown to watch the game outside on a big screen. There was a great sense of community on the streets. I was enjoying TEAMS more than any conference I had been to while working at Access Pass & Design. I felt much more comfortable in this environment of younger sports minded attendees.

TEAMS would usher in another partnership opportunity. I met a gentleman on the tradeshow floor who mentioned that if my intentions were to make a name in the professional sports industry, then I needed to meet the guy from the National Sports Forum, who was at the conference. "The guy's name is Dave Mullins, and I'll point him out if I see him or come grab you during the trade show if he's around."

While the TEAMS conference was geared toward tourism through sporting events, The National Sports Forum was all about professional sports and brought in teams from all of the professional sports leagues, such as Major League Baseball, the National Football League, the National Basketball Association, and the National Hockey League.

At the time my idea of working in the sports industry was everything that the National Sports Forum had to offer. I wanted to work with the big league teams. The following day, I left my booth unattended to introduce myself to Dave and said, "I would like to learn more about your event and if there is an opportunity, perhaps partner with you to provide the badges for it, much like we do for TEAMS."

Dave was interested and really liked our work. When he had time to visit my booth, he showed me a sample of what they had been using in the past. It was much flimsier than our badges and had more of a matte finish. It was functional but didn't have the flair and rigidity to compare to ours. Dave mentioned that another company had expressed interest in a badge partnership with the National Sports Forum and asked if I heard of a them. The company was called Cube and at the time they were our biggest competitor. That changed the entire tone of our conversation.

"Yes," I replied anxiously. "They're our biggest competitor."

Dave mentioned, "I have to give them first right of refusal but if our negotiations don't work out with them, then I'd love to give you a shot. I think your badges would make an excellent addition to our event."

I responded, "This is a golden opportunity, and I'll let you know right now that I want to do business with you. Just let me know what it's going to take."

Coincidently Dave and I were on the same shuttle bus back to the airport when the conference concluded. He needed to present the opportunity to the president of the National Sports Forum and gave the other company a deadline if they were in or out for the partnership. This was a contentious and exciting time, as I knew that locking in a deal with Dave would be the ultimate game changer for my career at Access Pass & Design.

Three weeks later Dave called me and asked if I was still interested in the deal.

"Definitely!"

"OK, then what I'll do is draft up an agreement for you to sign. You'll have rights to your logo on the badge, attendee database, mentions during the conference, and membership to the National Sports Forum Inner Circle." The deal was done within a week. In exchange, Access Pass & Design would provide the design services, and manufacture the badges and lanyards for the event. The biggest break of my career was meeting Lisa Furfine. The second biggest break was putting a deal together with the National Sport Forum.

The National Sports Forum, often referred to as the "Forum" is an annual three-day sports conference that traditionally takes place a week before the Super Bowl. Like TEAMS, it's held in a different city every year and showcases the best of what that city has to offer in terms of sports facilities and services. While TEAMS is more focused on tourism generated by sporting events, the National Sports Forum is more intensive on sales and marketing best practices, industry trends, insights, and economic issues.

My first Forum was held in Seattle at the end of January 2005. Dave Mullins introduced me to the president of The National Sports Forum, Ron Seaver. Ron expressed how much he loved the aesthetic look and feel of the badges that Access Pass & Design produced. At the 2005 Forum, held in Seattle, I connected with several executives from marketing agencies and sports properties within MLB, the NFL, the NHL, the NBA and even Churchill Downs racetrack. I was impressed by the prestige of the speakers and the sports facility site visits. We toured Quest Field, home of the Seattle Seahawks, and Safeco Field, home of the Seattle Mariners. The CEOs of each organization addressed the Forum at venue luncheons.

Seattle Seahawks CEO Tod Leiweke talked about the Hawks Nest in the north end zone. They are bleacher seats where the most rabid fans come to watch the game. They were his favorite seats, and he would often visit fans in the Hawks Nest during the game.

We also toured the University of Washington campus and athletic facilities. The athletic director presented a keynote speech on the last day of the Forum in one of the football hospitality suites.

But the keynote speech that blew me away was by Howard Schultz, CEO of Starbucks. He went half an hour over his allocated time slot, but no one seemed to mind. It seemed as if everybody wanted to stick around to hear him talk about the Starbucks business, Howard's tenacity, and the story of the brand. He was very much down to earth, connected to his employees, and very much involved with the community.

Access Pass & Design would enter a multiyear partnership agreement with the National Sports Forum, with first right of refusal, should we determine the event wasn't yielding a return. And with that deal, I was able to not only leverage the same benefits as the TEAMS conference but also a full-page color ad in the conference program. That was a big deal because no one else asked for it, and it was prime real estate. We'd get the back inside cover. Budweiser had rights to the back cover, the front cover was for the National Sports Forum, and the inside front cover was open for presenting sponsors.

My breakthrough year in the sports industry was in 2007. It was the year I landed my first deal with the New York Yankees, won the business of Texas Tech (who went on to win the Gator Bowl) and Illinois (who went on to The Rose Bowl), and established the company's highest grossing account.

The 2007 National Sports Forum was held in Los Angeles that year. The conference held a Budweiser Gala at Staples Center, where attendees received an exclusive VIP tour of the venue followed by a banquet dinner on the basketball court. Attendees were greeted by the Laker Girls.

After the Budweiser Gala conference attendees migrated to the hotel lobby bar at the National Sports Forum host hotel, the Hilton. I stayed until the bar closed at 2 a.m. and met some key contacts, one of whom was Matt Stoll from GMR Marketing. Also known as Stolli, Matt liked the quality of our work and the fact that we were partners with the National Sports Forum. He invited me to visit the GMR headquarters in New Berlin, Wisconsin, to meet the rest of their team.

While connecting with Matt was the key highlight for business opportunities, a breakout session hosted by Dan Migala revolutionized my way of thinking. Dan was a longtime alumni and steering committee member of the National Sports Forum. I never had a chance to meet him personally but had heard a lot of great things about his thought leadership in the industry.

The session Dan hosted was a series of case studies based on his personal consulting experience and real life observations. In 2006, 7-Eleven bought out a convenience store competitor and overnight increased its number of stores from 300 to 500. 7-Eleven presented a challenge to all of the Chicago-market professional sports organizations to help promote the recent acquisition. Whichever team presented the best idea would get the account.

Dan had a friend who worked for the Chicago White Sox, who called to inform him of the opportunity. They tossed around some ideas on traditional sponsorship, but nothing really stood out. Dan went out with some friends one night and was up later than he wanted to be, yet he still set his alarm clock for 7:30 a.m.

When he awoke, he stared at his alarm clock, and the time was 7:11. Dan swore it was 7:11 forever. So he called his guy at the White Sox and said, "We're going to buy six minutes of air time and change the game time from 7:05 p.m. to 7:11." The deal was done by noon that day.

The next story he told was one about the New York Marathon, which he also ran in 2006. He went on to ask the question, "Do your sponsorships enhance or interrupt the consumer experience?" As he ran the marathon, a herd of runners dressed in red ran past Dan, and one of them bumped into him. Shortly thereafter another herd dressed in red began to run past Dan, and he noticed that all of the runners were wearing AVIS Rent-A-Car shirts, that read We Try Harder.

Dan caught up to one of the runners and asked him what the big deal was, and the runner replied, "We have a sponsorship with the ING New York Marathon, and we're known as Achilles Heels runners. The person in the middle of this pack is blind."

That moment resonated with Dan, and he said to himself, "They get it."

Dan contacted the chief marketing officer of AVIS on Monday and asked him what the sponsorship was all about. "We didn't just want to sponsor the race, but we wanted to sponsor the emotion of what our brand was all about. We didn't buy physical inventory. We bought the moment that you had for yourself."

Everything Dan presented at the breakout session resonated. I redefined my perception of who I was in the industry, shifting from a sales executive to a marketer. At that point in my life, I had yet to run a marathon. I had been involved with *Team in Training* since 2000, and as an active participant I was a fund-raiser and participant for the century bike ride and completed an Olympic-distance triathlon. Between both events, I raised over $7,000 for the Leukemia & Lymphoma Society.

Dan's story about his experience at the New York Marathon ultimately inspired me to run the Nike Marathon later that year for *Team in Training*.

The 2007 National Sports Forum changed the way I did business. In fact, Access Pass & Design's return the 2007 Forum would result in 700% growth within a year.

To add, Ron Seaver was thrilled with our ongoing partnership and I asked him for a testimonial not long after the 2007 Forum. He came through big-time:

> *"When it comes to putting on conferences, one of the most important things to us is making that great first impression. And for us, that first impression begins and ends with Access Pass & Design. We are admittedly extremely finicky about how our name badges make us look— they have to be perfect. Which is why in our early years we used several different companies—but all that stopped when we started working with Access Pass & Design. Simply put, they get it. We're looking for professionalism, creativity, practicality, and visual appeal . . . and Access Pass & Design gives us ALL of that. We wouldn't work with anyone else."*

Summer of 2007 would be a whirlwind tour of capitalizing on opportunities in New York, Wisconsin, Illinois and San Francisco. At the end of July Brad Diller and I flew to Aurora, Illinois, to meet with the director of Super Cross, Dave Prater, along with his supervisor, Todd Jendro, for lunch. The following day we drove to New Berlin, Wisconsin to meet with Matt Stoll at GMR Marketing's headquarters. I worked with several people from their team earlier that year, so it was great to finally get a chance to meet them. Brad and I treated a group of 15 to lunch, and we bought ten tickets for the Brewers game at Miller Park that afternoon. GMR would become Access Pass & Designs highest grossing account over the next three years.

THE YANKEES - 2007, 2008

The highlight of the 2007 New York trip was definitely when I took my clients to two games at Yankee Stadium. The first game was against the Arizona Diamondbacks, where I brought a client, Shoop, who had sent me a nice piece of business earlier in the year. He was well connected and good friends with the Foo Fighters' tour manager at the time. My contact at the Yankees granted us press box access, where we watched a portion of the game. In the old Yankee Stadium, press box access meant that you could buy anything from the press box concession stand for one dollar. One dollar hot dogs, one dollar pizza slices, one dollar beers; it was grand. Right next to the concession stand was the organ player who plays the rally tunes during the game and in between innings. He was behind a pane of glass. Shoop and I always thought the music was pre-recorded, but we were watching the real deal playing the tunes right in front of us.

The game on the following day was game one of the Subway Series, the Yankees vs. the Mets. I brought along my two clients from AOL who had done a lot of business with Access that year: Jenny Stahl and Rachel Gross. We sat on the first tier up on the first base line, and Roger Clemens started that game. The stadium was sold out, and it got loud. We drank beers and had a blast!

2008 was the second year we worked with the Yankees, and it was also the final year of the old Yankee Stadium, "The House that Ruth Built." Access Pass & Design had an exceptional rapport with the organization and I kept in close contact with the media relations manager, Michael Margolis. A month before the final game, Michael asked if we would like to design a pass to commemorate the final game ever to be played at the old Yankee Stadium. Naturally, we did.

In December I would fly back to New York to attend the Motor Sports Marketing Forum, and was able to schedule another meeting with the Yankees and Michael Margolis. That meeting will forever rank in the top 10 all-time highlights of my career.

When I met with the Yankees, I received excellent treatment and compliments from the staff. The head security director told me, "You know I've been here for nearly 20 years, and I've seen a lot of credentials in my day. I don't tend to keep a lot of things, but the pass I received for the Yankees' final game is something I will take to my grave."

Michael ushered me on a personalized guided tour of the stadium, brought me onto the field, allowed me to sit in the dugout, and take as many pictures as I wanted. The only place I wasn't allowed to take pictures was in the Yankees locker room. I will admit that it was the best part of the tour and understood why I wasn't allowed to take pictures. It was hallowed ground. I remember seeing the lockers of Jeter, Rodriguez, Posada, Rivera, Giambi, Messina, Pettite, and Matsui. But the thing I remember the most about the locker room were the pillars that that were painted Yankee blue, with the NY logo carved in wood, painted white, and nailed to the pillars.

I had goose bumps not only in the locker room but also while sitting in the dugout and stepping in the batter's box, where greats like Mantle, Ruth, and DiMaggio swung their bats. I experienced firsthand the essence of a world-class organization with world-class tradition. Michael also provided world-class hospitality, and he was an ideal ambassador for the Yankees organization.

To commemorate the final year of the old Yankee Stadium, Access Pass & Design built a commemorative frame of the entire credential system for the 2008 season. On the bottom of the frame was a black and white photo of the opening from the old Yankee Stadium in 1923. Below that was a plaque of all the years they won the World Series, our logo, and a sentiment of appreciation for allowing Access Pass & Design to be a part of their history. That commemorative frame now lives in the New York Yankees media relations office.

CHAPTER 22
AN ENDURANCE LIFESTYLE

LIFE WITH TEAM IN TRAINING

During the cycling training season for Team in Training in 2004 I met a gentleman by the name of Boris Tavcar. His son, Zach, was diagnosed with Acute Lymphoblastic Leukemia in August of 2001 while he was a sophomore in high school. I was the first person Boris met who was remotely close to Zach's age. Boris got involved with the Leukemia & Lymphoma Society in 2003. He then joined Team in Training to raise awareness and money on his son's behalf.

I trained with the team and acted as an assistant cycling coach to Scott Robertson. Scott had been involved with the team for several years prior and was a highly accomplished marathoner and triathlete. Boris was a fan of Saturday Night Live and during some of our training rides, led by Scott, we'd talk like *The Ladies Man* and end every conversation with, "yeah, and dat's coo". But it wasn't until the evening before the 2004 AMBBR that we connected on several different levels.

Boris knew a thing or two about the music industry as he had been a drummer for a few bands, and was currently working back lighting at various venues around town. He also knew Seth Sheck. Boris heard bits and pieces of my story and thought of how unfair it was for a 23 year old who just graduated college to be diagnosed with brain cancer. Boris had a hard time accepting medical protocol, regimens, and statistics. Through Boris, I began to see things from my parents perspective. I was also reminded of the super intense emotional roller coaster from not only being a patient but what my parents had to go through as well.

Because of the steroids Zach would yell at Boris for no apparent reason, similar to how I yelled at my mom and dad while enduring treatment. Boris expressed how Zach was extremely passionate about playing high school football, and when cancer robbed him of his passion, Zach lost his anchor, much how I lost Europe. But the big difference between Zach and I was he was in his third year of treatment while my scans after 15 months of treatment, remained clean.

That night Boris questioned what my life was like before cancer. Did I live in an area with overhead power lines? Did my neighborhood have a high level of carcinogens? The only correlation between Zach and I is we grew up in virtually the same neighborhood, not even a half mile away from each other. But I had several other friends who lived just down the block from me and they never got sick. Our conversation helped put a lot of things into perspective for Boris given the difficulty of the process. We talked into the wee hours of the morning and got very little sleep that night. Boris would later describe the next day as follows:

As Scott came to the door and woke everyone up at 5am that morning, the darkness of the new day had quite a different feel. Rather than frustration and sadness there was an anticipated excitement. I remember rolling away from the start line and it was kind of nippy for a 5:30am on a summer day in Tahoe. Instead of this ride being a competitive event there was a feeling of calm and community.

I began to notice other Team in Training jerseys and will never forget a beautiful brunette woman who wore a picture of a very handsome young man on her jersey. She was riding by herself kind of away from her team but very melancholy. Older adult riders wore pictures of their children and it was then I realized this was a mass migratory movement of thought. People from all walks of life paying homage and sending energy to those still fighting this insidious disease.

As we climbed to the top of Emerald Bay to the first rest stop, the sun was starting to rise up over the mountains and it was incredibly beautiful; almost surreal that I was experiencing such beauty while my son and so many others experienced such pain. As the ride progressed I just remember this feeling of acceptance.

I got caught up in pedaling trying to keep up with you. I remember thinking to myself if this guy can kick my ass on those pedals then he will definitely be fine. From that point on I remember enjoying the ride and having some interesting conversations with folks. As we got to the finish line you were a bit ahead of me. When we crossed the finish line I remember looking for my son and giving him a big hug. I wanted to give him all the energy it took to do the ride and somehow magically bring and end to his process.

I handed him my number and thought everything happens for a reason. Maybe the reason was for him to be my teacher and show me how to live a better life. We introduced each other to our families, soon gathered our belongings, and said our goodbyes. The 2004 "America's Most Beautiful Bike Ride" was one of the most important and memorable experiences of my life! It allowed me to feel like I was giving back.

IF AT FIRST YOU DON'T SUCCEED, TRY TRI AGAIN

The sport of triathlon is an endurance challenge comprised of three disciplines: swim, bike, run. There are 4 classes of triathlons – sprint, Olympic or International, half Ironman, and full Ironman. A sprint typically consists of a .25 to .75 mile swim, 6 to 20 mile bike ride, and 2 to 5 mile run. An Olympic distance is a mile swim, 25 mile bike ride and 6.1 mile run. A half Ironman or 70.3 is a 1.2 mile swim, 56 mile bike, and 13.1 mile run. The granddaddy distance of all triathlon is an Ironman which is twice the distance of a half Ironman for a total of a 2.4 mile swim, 112 mile bike, and 26.2 mile marathon.

From 2002 to 2004 I competed in four triathlons. My first was the Donner Lake Sprint Triathlon in July 2002, and it took place a month after my first century (100-mile) bike ride around Lake Tahoe. I finished with a triathlon time of 1 hour, 5 minutes, 15 seconds. My time improved by nearly eight minutes in 2003 but fell back by nearly three minutes in 2004 with a time of 59 minutes, 53 seconds. 2005 was a breakthrough year for me in the sport of triathlon.

I loved the satisfaction of finishing a triathlon. Each race was a learning experience, as I discovered areas I could improve whether it was becoming stronger in one or two disciplines or becoming faster at each of my transitions. Transitions are when you move from one discipline to the next; T1 is swim to bike, T2 is bike to run. Although transitions only take minutes or even seconds, it could mean the difference between standing on the medal podium or in the crowd of admirers.

Traditionally there are overall award winners who are recognized with medals, plaques, or trophies at the end of every race. And they are gender-specific. The top three males and top three females are recognized. There are also age groups with winners that are broken down in five-year increments, with the exception of those who are 19 years old and younger. The top three finishers of each age group are awarded a position on the podium, and they are broken down as follows: 20-24, 25-29, 30-34, 35-39, 40-44, etc.

My Donner Sprint results in 2003 and 2004 could be improved with faster transition times and faster bike and run splits. And if I could figure out a way to improve my breathing technique during the swim and improve my transition times, I thought I would have pretty good chance to stand on that podium. There was good reason for me to aim for that goal.

The significance of the 2005 Donner Sprint for me was that I was 29 years old, and it was a way I could celebrate my fifth year of cancer remission. *How sweet would it be if I could win a spot on the podium that year?* Over the previous three years I observed how much faster and fit people were between the ages of 30 and 39. It's the most competitive age group, and if I didn't win a spot on the podium before entering that group, it might not be until my late fifties or sixties that I'd have another shot.

2005 was the first year that *Team in Training* had a Reno-Tahoe triathlon group. The target event would be the Pacific Grove triathlon, which was an Olympic-distance race. With my involvement and the friends that I made through TNT over the years, it was an easy decision for me. There were nearly twenty people who registered that year, and most were TNT marathon or cycling alumni.

Scott Robertson had been involved with *Team in Training* for nearly ten years in several capacities. He coached and participated in several marathons and century bike rides. Scott was the head cycling coach in 2003 and 2004, and in 2005 he would coach the first *Team in Training* triathlon group for the Reno-Tahoe area.

He was an exceptional endurance athlete whom I admired and looked up to. Up until 2005 he had also completed five Ironman Triathlons, including Ironman Lake Placid in 1999, Ironman Florida in 2000, Ironman Oceanside in 2001, and Ironman Canada in 2001 and 2002. His best Ironman finish time was 10 hours, 18 minutes in Florida. They were feats that I didn't yet realize or have the desire to achieve.

I met a guy by the name of Dave Fish in 2002, when Ann Conlin was the cycling coach for *Team in Training*. He was also a respectable athlete with multiple Ironman Triathlon achievements under his belt. He competed in the Cape Cod Iron distance events from 1983 through 1986, Ironman Florida in 1999, and Ironman Canada in 2004. In 2005 he was training for his second appearance in Ironman Canada and would also become the TNT swim coach.

Dave placed in countless endurance events over the years. In open water swims, he's about as fast as they get, with 2.4-mile Iron distance swim finishes under an hour, and on the bike course he's faster than most.

I already had a solid cycling base by the time I signed up for the Pacific Grove Triathlon, with the completion of the Chico Wildflower Century in April, the Indian Valley Century in May, and America's Most Beautiful Bike Ride in June.

Kelly Anderson recruited over 20 *Team in Training* participating

fundraisers to train for the Pacific Grove Triathlon. It was also the first organized group that I would train with under the guidance of Scott and Dave,
who were instrumental in our team's success. But my breakthrough happened during one of our first group swim workouts.

Dave supervised our swim workouts at the Double Diamond Athletic
Club, which donated pool hours for *Team in Training*. I was struggling with
my breathing during that first workout when Dave yelled from across the
pool, "Stop kicking, stop kicking! No wonder you're always tired in the
water. You're wasting all your energy."

When I finished that lap, he calmly explained, "You shouldn't be kicking much at all when you're swimming. Your stroke should be nice and
smooth. Your technique should be in the mechanics of your upper body. Try
getting across the pool without kicking this time."

The results were instant. I was much more fluid, calm and realized I had
a greater capacity to swim significantly longer by hardly any kicking at all.
When Liz Welsh and I enrolled in that swimming class in 2001, the instructor misled me. He continued telling me that I needed to kick as part of my
technique, but I could never figure out why I was always so tired. For nearly
five years I struggled with this. Dave Fish saved me.

The swimming revelation happened a month before the Donner Sprint
Triathlon, and my confidence skyrocketed. I felt so good about myself that I
registered for two more triathlons, including the Folsom Olympic Triathlon
and the Pyramid Lake Sprint once again.

Now that I had resolved my swimming issues, there was one element I
had no control over. When I raced the Donner Sprint from 2002 through
2004, I always experienced uncontrollable dizziness when exiting the water.
It was bad enough to the point I could not walk or run straight. It was something I had to battle through and take pause before getting on the bike. And
even when I was on the bike, it still took a few minutes for it to dissipate.

I finished the Donner Sprint with a time of 53 minutes, 16 seconds,
which was nearly four minutes faster than my previous personal record (PR)

in 2003. But was it fast enough to earn a position on the podium? The dizziness factor when I came out of the water was actually milder than it had been in previous years, but I struggled to remove my wetsuit, which cost me over a minute in transition and ultimately a third-place finish. I would finish seventh overall out of 46 in my age group.

The field for my age group that year seemed particularly fast. The third-place finishing time was 50 minutes, 20 seconds, which is a time I couldn't beat even if I shaved two minutes from my finishing time. But after analyzing where I could've improved, I was very happy with my result as a milestone achievement for my 5th year of remission. A year later I learned that my 2005 time would have earned me a third place in the 24–29 age division. As the saying goes, "Timing is everything."

The first triathlon *Team in Training* group for the Reno-Area would raise nearly $60,000 in 2005 for the Leukemia & Lymphoma Society. Scott and Kelly praised our team with an e-mail:

SCOTT

Thanks to everyone who came out yesterday and celebrated Reno TNT Triathlon Team #1. Thanks to all of you dedicated and positive athletes who participated in a fun and rewarding season. You raised lots of $ for the LLS. Thanks to Dave [Fish], many of you improved your swimming skills and learned to swim in the open water. Thanks, great mentors Liz and Liana. Thanks for TNT support from Kelly.

What's next? As alumni you are welcome to come out to the workouts, and I will keep you on the e-mail list. Of course we hope to have you come out and help newbies with the ropes. Some of you are interested in competing in Vineman 70.3 next year, so I will be sending out information on when to sign up, and of course we'll have a workout schedule for that too.

See you soon.—Scott

KELLY

Thank YOU Scott!! You did an outstanding job coaching us throughout the season! Our tri team raised just shy of $60,000!! Way to Go! Thank you for your determination and dedication!

I look forward to seeing you all out on some runs and rides before the weather turns yucky!

Take care —Kelly

SIX YEARS WITH TNT

2006 was also my sixth year of affiliation with *Team in Training*. The acting cycling coach in 2004 and 2005 decided to move on, and I was interested in taking the position. Before I could express my interest, Kelly Anderson asked if I wanted to take the role. With my four years of experience, dedication, and honor-patient history with TNT, I was the unanimous candidate. Kelly offered the position in the spring of 2005, and after AMBBR that year, I attended a coaching certification course at Mont Bleu, a casino resort in south Tahoe.

Scott Robertson helped me out tremendously in my first year and shared much of his past racing and coaching experience. He stated in an e-mail, "Next, I hope to assist Danny Heinsohn with the spring cycling team. I know from coaching that team that more assistance is needed, particularly on long rides when you need to keep track of riders that can be separated by several miles. I would like to help with the recruiting meetings as well as the seminars and workouts."

From 2006 through 2008, I would lead three *Team in Training* cycling groups to cross the finish line from a century bike ride. Roughly forty would complete the training, and the cumulative total in fundraising by all exceeded $125,000 for the Leukemia & Lymphoma Society. The lifelong friendships I made along the way will forever be cherished.

2007 - THE MARATHON CHALLENGE

My first weekend off in 2007 didn't come until the first weekend of November. If I wasn't travelling for work, I would be training for my next triathlon and coaching the *Team in Training* cycling group for AMBBR, or attending Mark Wood's bachelor party and wedding. I competed in the Wildflower Triathlon Olympic distance that year. After AMBBR in June, business travel took me to Dallas for 5 days followed by 10 days in New York.

While in New York, I was relaxing in my hotel room and realized I had no business trips between the end of July and mid-October. I decided to sign up for the Nike Women's Marathon for my third fundraising initiative with *Team in Training*. Dan Migala's story at the New York Marathon and the AVIS activation inspired me to make that decision.

Team in Training in Reno would not have been the success that it was, had it not been for the dedication of Ski Pisarski. Since August 1995 Ski coached over 25 teams for the *Team in Training* and ran over 100 marathons throughout his life. He spent time in the military and he gained weight when he got out. Ski resorted to running as a means to stay healthy and keep the weight off.

Throughout his tenure he inspired and helped train hundreds in the Reno area, directed over 30 local racing events, ran 17 Boston Marathons, 20 California Internationals, 24 Napas, 1 Ultra Marathon, and over 300 shorter distance races. He was the godfather of our local *Team in Training* group. Ski was eternally optimistic and always in a good mood. When I became an honored patient for the *Team in Training* in 2000, Ski treated me like a grandkid and always offered his assistance. His motto to everyone was *Keep Smilin'.*

I didn't enjoy running as much as I liked to cycle. Year after year he would ask me, "When are you going to train for a marathon? We will welcome you any time you're ready."

But I made a promise to Ski that I would train for a marathon while he led the *Team in Training* group; it was only a matter of when.

The year 2007 was already a whirlwind, with all of my business adventures, cycle team coaching, and triathlon training. *Team in Training* was the charitable beneficiary of the Nike Women's Marathon, slated to take place in San Francisco on October 17. The Nike Women's Marathon was also open to men who and primarily marketed to those who were a part of *Team in Training.*

There was a two-month gap between my business trips leading up to the race. I was already conditioned from my cycling and triathlon training; all I needed to do was focus my energy on running. Upon my return from a ten day business trip in New York, I made the commitment to run the race and to raise money for the Leukemia & Lymphoma Society for a third time.

Most everyone from *Team in Training* in the Reno Area knew who I was because of my involvement as cycling coach, but I did not know many of the runners. The Reno TNT running group was about 80-strong at the time, and we filled the streets whenever we ran together. The standard group runs were on Tuesdays at 6 p.m. and Saturday mornings at 7 a.m. We had a strong backbone of TNT alumni/mentors who were instrumental in the success of the group. Everyone was vested in the success of everyone else, and it was awesome to be a part of that synergy. The mentors were always available for support via phone, e-mail, or on the training runs themselves. In fact *Team in Training* at the time was one big happy family, in Reno.

It was really nice to be back on the participant side. All I had to do was show up to the workouts and run. The mentor support during my time of training was phenomenal and many of them were Boston Marathon finishers. Sara Holmes and Daryn Carns were my assigned mentors. Christy Lew, Andy Szeto, Elizabeth Welsh, and Stephanie Wilch were also amazing runners and mentors who were always there to support and motivate the first-time marathoners. Ski was the head coach, and Eric Beyes was the speed-training coach.

Week in and week out we'd train as a group. Tuesday nights we'd focus on running speed intervals, while Saturdays were meant to achieve breakthrough mileage. The last two miles of any breakthrough mileage run always seemed to be the toughest. The longest we trained as a group was 22 miles and that was three weeks before the marathon.

At the pasta feed on marathon eve, I learned that the national effort of *Team in Training* raised over $18 Million for the Leukemia & Lymphoma Society as all participants trained for the Nike Women's Marathon.

I would go on to finish the marathon with the fastest time in our group that year at exactly four hours. And with the marathon finish I would become a *Team in Training* Triple Crowner. What that means is I competed in all three of Team in Training's endurance events which included a 100 mile century bike ride, an Olympic distance triathlon, and a full marathon. Along the way, I exceeded the fundraising minimums for each event for a grand total of over $12,000 for the Leukemia & Lymphoma Society.

CHAPTER 23

PUTTING EVERYTHING TOGETHER

2009 - REALIZING THE IRONMAN DREAM

The first year I attended the National Sports Forum was in 2005. Dave Mullins introduced me to Bonner Paddock, who was the director of sponsorships for the Forum. Bonner was always very genuine, energetic, and sincere. A month following the conference in 2005, he began a five-year career with the Anaheim Ducks and was the senior manager of corporate partnerships. The Ducks would win the Stanley Cup in 2007. And in 2009 Bonner would inspire me to go beyond my limits.

The National Sports Forum was held in Phoenix, Arizona, in 2009. Kevin Lyman, founder of Van's Warped Tour, was on a panel discussion called the "Blending of Sports and Entertainment." Van's Warped Tour had been a client of Access Pass & Design since we opened in 2002, so it was interesting to see a music veteran speak on a sports panel.

Bud Selig, the commissioner of Major League Baseball, and NHL legend Wayne Gretzky were also keynote speakers. When Bud Selig finished his talk on the state of Major League Baseball, the lights went out, the jumbo screens on both sides of the podium lit up, and a documentary began to roll.

It was a trailer that began with the legs of a man hiking with a pigeon-toed limp. It was Bonner. The opening dialogue began in Bonner's voice. "I don't see how there's any way of making it to the top if I'm this tired already. Kilimanjaro is a tough climb, but for me it will be tougher with cerebral palsy."

Oscar-nominated actor Michael Clarke Duncan picked up the narration with, "This is Bonner Paddock. Bonner developed cerebral palsy when he was deprived of oxygen during birth. To climb Kilimanjaro, he will hurdle through an oxygen-thin challenge of his own creation."

Bonner had a friend whose son passed away from cerebral palsy at a very young age. His name was Jake, and Bonner vowed to do everything in his power to ensure this would not happen to another child with a disability. The trailer lasted for two minutes and concluded with Bonner standing on the top of Mt. Kilimanjaro.

The closing narration was the voice of Michael Clarke Duncan, "Through the freezing cold. Through thin air. Beyond limits."

When the trailer ended and the lights were illuminated, there wasn't a dry eye in the room. Ron Seaver introduced Bonner Paddock, and the room erupted with cheers and a standing ovation. Bonner revealed that he founded an organization named OM Foundation, a nonprofit to build centers for disabled children in Africa and the United States. OM stands for One Man, One Mission. I was truly inspired, and in the back of my mind, I began to think that 2010 would be my tenth year of brain cancer remission. *What could I do to celebrate that milestone?*

Coaching *Team in Training* was rewarding because I could see firsthand how the process changed peoples' lives and instilled confidence. Finishing a first marathon, triathlon or century bike could be a life defining moment to some. It certainly was for me.

2008 was my last year of involvement with *Team in Training*. It was time to take a break after nearly nine years. I really enjoyed coaching, but soon realized I was also holding myself back from my full potential of being an endurance athlete. I wanted to excel and take my training to a new level.

I competed in the Escape from Alcatraz Triathlon in June 2009 and had the time of my life. Later that summer, I put more thought into how I would celebrate my ten-year remission from brain cancer. July 19, 2010, would be the ten-year mark since my final month of chemo. I contemplated how I could top my accomplishments from *Team in Training*. Should I raise money for Livestrong, or *Team in Training* again, or start my own initiative? Who would I train with? What race should I do?

I began to think about my early years in cycling with *Team in Training* and the people I looked up to. I reflected and remembered those who were accomplished Ironman finishers. Dave Fish, Scott Robertson, and Jessica Eisenberg—each had a resume of Ironman finishes. I rode with them from time to time during my tenure with *Team in Training*. Ironman Canada was the event they trained for when I first became acquainted with them. Dave Fish once told me that Ironman Canada was his favorite race for several reasons, but the one thing I remember in particular was the time of year it took place. Ironman Canada took place at the end of August every year, which was great timing for me. Historically most of my business travel ended in June and didn't start up again until mid-September or later.

Dave and Scott were my advocates from that point forward. I began to research Ironman Canada and leaned on them for insights. Most Ironman bike courses have two or more loops around the same route, which makes it spectator friendly. But one of the unique features of Ironman Canada is its one-loop bike course with two big hills. That's right, one 112-mile loop. They mentioned that the hills on the bike course were very similar in distance and profile to a few of the lofty hill climbs we regularly trained on in the Reno-Tahoe area. Ironman Canada was also one of the most challenging bike courses in the Ironman series.

Some of the popular races in the Ironman series sell out in a matter of 24 hours or less. Canada, Lake Placid, and Arizona were among the most popular. There is an online process to register for any Ironman event, except for Ironman Kona, which to my knowledge was by invitation, qualifying time, or a few lucky lottery slots. Based on Scott and Dave's input, Ironman Canada is known for selling out in the first day from both on-site and online registrations. But they've never turned anyone down if they registered on-site.

I had every reason to train for Ironman Canada to celebrate the decade milestone of being free from brain cancer. The fact that my 10th year of remission happened to fall in 2010 truly made this a once-in-a-lifetime opportunity, and I didn't take it lightly. I determined that it was time to train for an Ironman triathlon. I resolved to make the trek to the event in Penticton, BC, at the end of August 2009 and register for the 2010 competition in-person.

Penticton is the town where Ironman Canada begins and ends, and is an approximate 3.5 hour drive from Vancouver, BC. The town itself has a growing population, of roughly 40,000. Ironman Canada had been a staple in the community for nearly 30 years and was a vital to Penticton's tourism economy. In fact over 4,000 people in the town's community volunteered annually for the Ironman event.

I reserved a camp spot at Wright's RV Park prior to leaving for Canada. When I arrived, the park was nearly full and I came to find out that many of the surrounding campers in RV's were in preparation for the race. I met a woman named Michelle Morck at the campground's general store, and she was from the greater Seattle area. We talked about how we each drove from Seattle to register for the 2010 race. She drove up with her husband, Brian, who was at their campsite when she introduced me to him.

We visited each other intermittently throughout the weekend to talk about why we each decided to train for an Ironman, and also about life in general. Over recent years Michelle participated in a handful of short distance triathlons and one half Ironman event. She was now ready for the personal challenge of training for a full Ironman. We would exchange contact information and stay in touch to support each other over the next year.

During the weekend of Ironman Canada I also scouted surrounding hotels and placed reservation holds on two of them. Dave Fish recommended I do this as the best vacancies fill up quickly. Although I would've preferred a hotel close to the race start, it simply wasn't affordable at nearly $300 to $500 per night. Months later I decided to finalize reservations with the Carmi Motor Inn, which had a kitchen and two bedrooms. It was less than five miles away from the race start.

FOR A REASON

One of my first contacts at GMR Marketing was an account director for MillerCoors in the North Carolina, Maryland, and Georgia regions. I began working with Tiffany Baird in 2006. She gave me a glowing testimonial in 2007, after Access Pass & Design had exceeded and delivered beyond all of her expectations:

> *Danny has been an amazing client services rep for me over the past few years on every project we have worked on. He is always responsive to my calls and e-mails and works hard to give multiple product options as well as solutions that meet our budget parameters. His integrity, both with his work and the causes he's associated with, is unmatched. His work ethic and passion are contagious on many levels. You will truly enjoy your experience working with Danny.*

Tiffany later introduced me to her husband, Brian Gross. Brian was the director of event marketing and hospitality for Roush Fenway Racing, and over the years I became pretty good friends with both. Then in 2009, Brian contacted me and mentioned that he was working with Livestrong on some marketing initiatives. In July he invited me to the Celebrity Golf Tournament at Edgewood in South Lake Tahoe.

After all these years I had never been to the Celebrity Golf Tournament, although I had been aware of the star power that the event attracted, including regulars such as Michael Jordan, Charles Barkley, Jerry Rice, and John Elway. I had the privilege to watch Jordan, Rice, and Ray Allen play as a threesome that year.

Brian knew I was on a mission to celebrate my ten years of brain cancer remission, and I leaned on him for his business development and marketing expertise to help me get started. I wanted to create an organization called Hometown Heroes, which was a name inspired by those who were there for me during my time in the hospital, and throughout chemotherapy.

They were my heroes who inspired me to keep fighting, and with that came an eternally optimistic outlook. Brian looked into the URL, and it was already claimed. Then about a week later he called to inform me that www. myhometownheroes.org was available. It was a better fit because if anyone were to ever say "My" they are claiming ownership. It had a good ring to it and I purchased the domain name immediately.

PRELIMINARY TRAINING

Upon my return from a Yosemite vacation after the Labor Day holiday weekend, I registered for the Las Vegas Marathon, which would take place on December 6. That gave me nearly three months to prepare. My finish time at my first marathon in 2007 was 4 hours on a hilly course. I set my sights on a 3:45 finish time on the Las Vegas flat course. This would be a great opportunity to establish my base training for Ironman Canada.

Coach Ski started a new endurance training group in 2008 called Northern Sierra Endurance Training (NSET), and the majority of all *Team in Training* alumni migrated along with him, including me. I trained in the usual fashion with the NSET running group with progressively longer runs on Saturday mornings and faster short-distance runs on Tuesday evenings. Now that my training regimen was established, I refocused on my pursuits to tie a charity initiative back into my ten-year remission. It was then that I decided to approach a couple of business-minded friends whom I thought would make great partners to form an initiative.

My friends, Brian Kuykendall and Dan Carlstrom were 100 percent onboard. Seth Sheck of Access Pass & Design was also on-board. On Tuesday, November 24, the four of us were able to meet for lunch at the El Adobe Café to sit down and brainstorm. My opening comments with Brian, Dan, and Seth were, "I would like to form a fund-raising initiative that I can tie into my training for Ironman Canada with the goal of raising $10,000 to symbolize 10 years of brain cancer remission."

My initial thoughts were to raise money for local families that were going through treatment and in need of financial aid or trying to recover financially from medical expenses. Although Brian, Dan, and Seth liked the idea, they thought it should be more condensed and specific.

Brian mentioned, "Why don't you create a scholarship fund for cancer survivors?"

Dan and Seth thought it was a great idea, and it was decided that My Hometown Heroes would be a scholarship fund for young cancer survivors.

I finished the Las Vegas Rock n' Roll Marathon on the first weekend of December with a time of 3 hours, 41 minutes, four minutes faster than my goal time. I was satisfied, plus my mom and dad were there to cheer me on.

Access Pass & Design's Christmas bonuses would be issued at the company's holiday party a couple of weeks following the marathon. I decided to use my bonus to finance the start-up costs of My Hometown Heroes. A consultant recommended that I add "Inc." to the official name. So in January of 2010, My Hometown Heroes, Inc., was approved by the Secretary of State of Nevada to operate as a local nonprofit organization.

CHAPTER 24

DECADE MILESTONE

"The two most important days of your life are the day you are born and the day you find out why."
—Mark Twain

SCARRED FOR LIFE

Brain cancer didn't kill me. It made me stronger and more resilient. However, the scar tissue that resulted from the removal of my tumor would leave me prone to seizures for the rest of my life. The risk factors were greatest when I trained longer and harder, or when I travelled for work.

The combination of flying two to three time zones away, losing sleep, and staying out late to network was a recipe for a seizure. I learned that I would have to double my dose of anti-seizure meds to stay in the safety zone; but I wasn't always faithful to that protocol. Often times the networking opportunities were so good that I simply forgot to take my meds. I never had a seizure when I travelled with Seth because our travels were always in the same time zone. But there were incidences when I was in New York and Chicago that caused me to miss hours of networking time.

First I could sense my mind begin to race with repetitive thoughts. I learned to combat an oncoming seizure by reciting songs in my head. That was my primary line defense if I hadn't taken my meds. But once that line of defense was down, I'd instantly lose my ability to speak, and I would soon get the head spins. Sometimes my entire body would become numb and transcend into a state of intense vertigo.

But it wasn't business trips that stressed my body out to the point of having a seizure. There were incidences when I trained with *Team in Training* that I would have to pull over on my bike and someone else from the group would call for a vehicle to pick me up. Business, endurance training, and preventing seizures were all a part of my survivorship lifestyle.

MAN ON A MISSION

At the age of 34, in my tenth year of remission from brain cancer, I lived a lifetime.

Needless to say, my number one priority of 2010 was to train for Ironman Canada and get My Hometown Heroes off the ground. I designed my training schedule to allow me to work normal business hours Monday through Friday. Training workouts would take place early in the morning, during lunch, or after I left the office.

Business travel would take me to Los Angeles for client meetings at the beginning of January, the National Sports Forum in Baltimore at the end of January, Chicago for the IEG sponsorship conference in mid-March, and the Event Marketing Summit during the first week of May. Beyond that, my next business trip wasn't scheduled until the Sports Sponsorship Symposium, held in New York, a few weeks following my big race. This meant I would have nearly four uninterrupted months of training without the toll that work travel took on my immune system.

I planned for three half Ironman distance events in consecutive months beginning with the Auburn Long Course on May 23, also known as the "Worlds Toughest Half Iron Distance." Boise 70.3 would take place three weeks later on June 12, and a repeat appearance at Vineman 70.3 would occur on July 18. Up until this point I only competed in one half Ironman race, and that was back in 2006. Ironman Canada would take place on Sunday, August 29.

With the assistance of my creative director at Access, Bill Nutt, we created a My Hometown Heroes website through Word Press. I then created a Facebook fan page and Twitter handle to get the word out and to make milestone announcements. For example May 17 was the day I was diagnosed in 1999, and July 19 was my last day of chemo in 2000.

To stay engaged, I also planned to post my race results on Facebook, and I developed a MHH fund-raising website. The goal was to raise $10,000 to reflect ten years of brain cancer remission.

Above all 2010 was planned as a year of celebration and reflection on a decade of being cancer-free. I wanted to acknowledge, inspire, and give thanks to everyone who had been a part of my life since the day I was diagnosed to the present.

JANUARY – THE OFFICIAL LAUNCH OF MY HOMETOWN HEROES

On January 3, 2010, I made my tenth-year remission milestone and Ironman Canada announcement "Facebook official":

> *To celebrate my 10 years of cancer survivorship in 2010, I'm building a scholarship fund for young cancer survivors, coaching and mentoring athletes for cycling and triathlons, competing in three half Ironman triathlons, leading up to the grand finale to compete in Ironman Canada on August 29, all while working with the biggest names in sports and entertainment.*

The responses and "likes" were immediate and abundant:

> *You kicked cancer's butt, which already makes you an Ironman in my book. Any help I can offer you for your efforts, just let me know! You definitely are an inspiration.*

> *I can't believe it's been ten years! I remember staying at the hospital with you! Congrats & you're amazing & thoughtful for giving back!*

> *Wow! I find your efforts very inspiring. I lost my father to cancer nearly 20 years ago. Thanks for giving back to cancer survivors.*

Danny, you are an inspiration to all of us! Let me know what I can do to help.

WOW, I had no idea. I lost my mother to cancer in '07 and my father in '06. It ripped our family apart, but then it made us stronger. Learning what can cause cancer, such as food and environment, we changed. I can only pray that it won't hit our family again. With surviving something that vicious, you can survive anything! Have a great tenth-year celebration!

I exercised all of my resources to share my story, including the team at Access Pass & Design, my clients, the National Sports Forum, TEAMS network, NSET, local media, friends, and family.

At the end of January I was back at the National Sports Forum, this time in Baltimore. Bill Nutt was a huge sports fan, and I wanted him to experience the event and learn how business gets done in the industry.

The 2010 show was a record breaker in attendance and in my opinion had the most high-profile panel lineup of speakers at any conference I had been to. One of the keynote panels included Cal Ripken Jr., the CEO of Feld Entertainment, the CEO of Under Armour, and Ted Leonsis, majority owner of the Washington Capitals.

I was in the zone and overly excited about meeting with old Forum friends and networking with new peers, including the corporate marketing officer of the UFC (Ultimate Fighting Championship) and the global brand manager of EA Sports. In the midst of that excitement, I neglected to take my anti-seizure medication. During the middle of the Inner Circle luncheon, I began to feel a seizure coming on, so I stood up, walked out of the room, and headed for the elevator which was nearly a football field length down the hall.

The seizure was overwhelming. My ability to speak was lost, my arms and hands became numb, and I began to get head spins. I honestly thought I could make it to the elevator and back to my room without confrontation.

I made it to the elevator and reached to my back pocket to grab my wallet where I stowed my hotel room key. That was as far as I got.

There seemed to be a motor disconnection in my arm. I could not find my back pocket to grab my wallet. The next thing I knew, my friend Preston Carter saw me sitting by the elevator with my hand on my head. He asked if I was all right, and I shook my head no. Soon Bonner came around the corner and found out that I was having a hard time. They informed the conference coordinator and Ron Seaver, and they were able to track down Bill Nutt, who arrived a few minutes later. Bill and Bonner were somewhat familiar with my medical condition.

I was soon escorted to a side room with a couple of the hotel concierges, who were helpful. I was grateful for everyone's help, which was reflective of the family spirit that the Forum fosters. Eventually Bill walked me back up to my hotel room, where I slept for nearly four hours.

I had built a lot of networking momentum during the first two days of conference and looked forward to attending the Budweiser Gala that was hosted by the Baltimore Ravens. I unfortunately missed it, but Bill was able to enjoy the experience without me.

The seizure was one of the worst I can recall and could have been prevented, had I stayed current with my medication. Business travel and the networking activities that go along with it are taxing enough. But with a seizure condition like mine, it takes a higher toll, and I usually need to increase my dosage of the medication. In this case I failed to do both and suffered the consequences. After the Forum I returned to Reno with Bill safe and sound, and I decided to not inform my parents of the incident.

ROAD TO IRONMAN CANADA

My training didn't have the continuity I had hoped for after I completed the Rock n' Roll Marathon in December. I continued to instruct my spinning class on Thursday evenings, but I kept my running to a minimum. Due to a long winter my miles for January were fewer than I had hoped for; they also would have been more had it not been for my business trips to LA and Baltimore. I wasn't too concerned, but I really wanted to push 200 miles in February and 300 in March. Business travel would always set me back a couple of weeks, so I wanted to be on the aggressive side with the mileage whenever possible.

Despite my commitment of training for Ironman Canada, I had a pretty cohesive game plan to drive sales at Access Pass & Design and also to launch a fund-raising initiative for My Hometown Heroes. At the beginning of the year, I informed a few of my friends in the fitness community that I wanted to start an annual charity run to benefit My Hometown Heroes. It would take place on the first day of spring, and I thought about calling it the Spring Into Action 5k.

Dave Fish got back to me and suggested I contact Ryan Ress, owner of Reno Running Sports, an online listing of local running events. Coincidently he was also planning a community run on the same day. Ryan was one of the fastest runners in town, and he had prior race director and course development experience. He contacted me first:

Danny-

I was talking to Dave Fish, and he mentioned you wanting to put on a spring race. I was trying to find out what day you had planned on doing that. I'm putting together one at Cottonwood Park on March 20th, Spring Day. If you had planned on the same day, I would be more than happy to partner up with NSET, if you wanted to be a part of the Reno Running Event. My permits are already in. Let me know.

Thanks,

Ryan

While Ryan was the race director, I was in charge of sponsorship sales for T-shirts and banner ads. We put the race together in less than three months, and despite a major unforeseen circumstance on my end, we still managed to register over 125 participants. Spring Into Action made a total of over $4,000 between sponsorship sales and registration fees. After city permit fees, an on-site EMT, and basic race supplies, we still made a net profit of over $3,000, which we split. My portion went directly to My Hometown Heroes.

January Training Mileage:
4.5 Swim, 56 Bike, 54.5 Run
TOTAL: 115

FEBRUARY – YOU CAN'T EXPECT THE UNEXPECTED

Research has led experts to believe that cancer may be attributed to various outside factors, including, genetics, environment, diet, habits, and lifestyle. It's easy to look back and consider what element or combination of elements may lead to my diagnosis. Through education, research, and awareness it can be prevented or the risk greatly reduced.

Along the same lines life has a way of testing our capacity beyond prevention. Living through brain cancer and thriving through endurance training has taught me timeless life lessons. One of those is that you can't expect the unexpected. And when the unexpected happens, you can only choose how to deal with it.

When I returned home from the National Sports Forum, I called my dad to let him know how much of a success the trip had been. I always called him with good news, and he was always glad to hear it. I bragged about the possibility of working with the UFC.

My birthday followed the day after I returned from Baltimore, on Friday, February 5. I invited several friends and my parents to my house for a potluck celebration that Saturday evening. Valentine's Day landed on a Sunday, and I had dinner with my parents that night. It seemed like a normal night, but I found it somewhat peculiar that my dad was unusually quiet. I didn't venture to ask him if anything was wrong, but I had a premonition. Just before I left, I put my hand on his shoulder while he sat in front of the computer and said, "Love you, Dad. I'll see you tomorrow."

Without warning or any other relevant signs, my dad passed away the next evening.

Comprehension of this unexpected event was far beyond me and goes far beyond words. Everyone in our lives was devastated and in complete shock. In the wee hours of the following morning, I woke up crying my eyes out as I lie next to my mom. We cried all night.

Family, friends, and his coworkers poured their love and support to honor his memory. They flew or drove into town the next few days, and the funeral and wake would be held the following Saturday. I was numb and in shock the entire first week, as I worked tirelessly with my mom to prepare everything.

This period of time reminded me somewhat of the busyness after being diagnosed with cancer—so many affairs to line up, including paperwork, family schedules, acting as a center hub of communication, ready to take action and help the cause at any time. This time I was on the receiving end. It was what my dad did for me and what I would do for him. Nothing was more important at that time than honoring his legacy.

I thought I knew my father through and through. He was my dad. But over the next few days, I learned a lot more about him through his friends, family, and coworkers. At the funeral everyone had something special to say. My cousins Windy and Michael and I agreed to present our speech together at the funeral service, but we would discuss different memories. I commented on our time at the hospital at UCLA, about constipation, *Saturday Night Live* skits, and ridiculous songs he'd sing out of key when he woke me up in the morning as a kid.

While the funeral was a quiet time for mourning and reflection with family and a few of his coworkers, the wake provided an opportunity for friends and coworkers to express their regards. Most of my training peers, the owners and a few team members of Access Pass & Design, personal friends, and a few of my mom's friends from church visited to express their condolences. I learned later that night of the dozens of cars that wrapped around the entire block.

FROM A COWORKER

From different perspectives I learned a lot about my dad and was reminded of how caring, trusting, and loyal he was during his life. In the office he was known as "The Rock." As a veteran IT specialist who worked for the State of Nevada, he was the most robust problem solver of the group, and they could always count on him. One of his coworkers sent an e-mail the day following the service:

Danny,

As I mentioned yesterday at the service, I only knew your dad for a short time (May 2008). When I first got hired, he helped get me set up with the things people don't think about. He gave me a good spreadsheet for keeping track of my time. Got me going in our little coffee club. It was just three of us until recently. He would buy the worst coffee sometimes, and Donna and I used to razz him about it, and next time he'd find something even worse. It's become funny to me. We shared a love of Subarus and talked cars quite a bit. My pop also loved cars. When Ted and I talked about cars, I'd look at him, and it reminded me of my dad, and I'd smile to myself about it. He was usually in the lead when we walked. He'd change into his walking shoes and sometimes I'd say, "Come on, Old Man, get your slippers on." (I used to call my dad either Pop or Old Man.) I just recently started to see his silly bone that you talked about. I had no idea he even went to a casino until recently. I asked him, and he said Tamarack Junction was his place. I listen to the radio all day long, and that jingle in their commercial would come on and I'd try to sing it to him: "Taaamarack Junction, your junction for fun!" Then he'd sing one from a different casino.

This is when I started to discover his silly bone. As necessary, we have to keep it hidden at work for the most part. I love the lightness of silly. I was lucky enough to be born with one. I think the silly bone is a DNA thing, and I'm sure you have it, too. The world needs more silly. My younger sis and I were talking about this not long ago. She's also fortunate enough to have the gift of silly. I wish I'd have discovered his sooner, but in my area it's been crazy busy since the day I got hired.

I lost my dad to cancer in 2004 and my mom to just wearing down in 2007. Like one of your buds on FB mentioned, it does get better with time, but the key word is better. It took me a long time to get healed enough to function properly after my folks passed. I can say that there will be times that something will remind me, and I'll have a short cry. Some folks don't understand and think crying is weak or bad or whatever. I think concerning the tears over my folks, it's more of a gift. They loved me so much, they gave me the gift to love others; and where there is love, the losses are heartfelt, hence the crying.

I will also say that you will probably find yourself forgetting things here and there in the coming months. Go easy on yourself, as it's normal. Your brain will also be looping whether you like it or not, and the details of life will now and again get lost in the shuffle. I once got out of my car to meet a buddy and left my car running with the doors locked! It sat in that parking lot and idled for two hours. These are the little things that could happen, so again, go easy on yourself. I can't stress it enough. We all deal differently, but those who try to just work through the pain don't get the gifts the pain brings. Gifts of what's important, what isn't, etc. It's hard to put your finger on, but they are gifts. Feel it and move a step forward. Repeat as necessary. (Could be six months, could be two years.) You've been through a lot already, and I'm sure I'm not telling you anything you don't already know.

I don't know what else to say, but you now have my e-mail, and if you ever need anything, don't hesitate to write me.

Love,

Scott Russel

FROM A CHILDHOOD FRIEND

One of my dad's childhood friends, Bob Ellefson, still lived in Southern California, where my dad grew up. When Bob moved to Northridge as a kid, he didn't know anyone. Bob and my dad met while fooling around in the street and said hi to each other. Soon they were playing football and baseball in the middle of the street.

Bob was somewhat of a home-body, and my dad was an outdoorsy guy who loved to hunt and fish. He got Bob into those things. Back then in the late 1950s, the San Fernando Valley had a lot of rural areas, so they would shoot crows with bows and arrows and as they got older would hunt pheasants in the San Joaquin Valley.

My dad was the kind of guy who would call Bob and say, "Let's go fishing."

My dad exposed Bob to deep-sea fishing in Coos Bay, and they would take their catches to a cannery to smoke them on-site. As they drove home, they couldn't wait, so they opened up the cans of smoked salmon and ate them as they drove back to Southern California.

When Bob and my dad were in high school, they ran a poker club once a month when the parents weren't home. Bob says my dad really got into it. What they enjoyed most was the camaraderie within their group of friends and telling stories of crazy things. One time someone brought cigars, and everyone was choking after they lit up.

Bob was living with his parents during his first year of college and was dating his future wife, Irene. My dad called Bob one day and said, "We gotta go to Las Vegas. Come on, it will be a lot of fun." Back then, the airlines were only charging $10 each way.

Ted asked Bob, "You got a credit card, right?"

"Yeah, with a $100 limit."

Bob called Irene to tell her he was sick. They flew down to play the 21 tables and lost all of their money. They were stranded without a flight home and no way back to the airport. They carried bags for elderly people for tips until they had enough money to get a cab back to the airport.

They went to a lot of Dodger games at the L.A. Coliseum before Chavez Ravine. In particular they'd go to games when Sandy Koufax and Don Drysdale pitched. They collected hoards of baseball cards and built their own skateboards out of roller skates for hobbies.

I asked Bob how things were with my dad when I was diagnosed with cancer. It was life-or-death, panic, and urgency—but there was a lot of hope. Bob could sense fear in my dad's voice the way he said things. As time went on through my treatment, my dad would inform close friends such as Bob and their mutual childhood friend, Phil Norton, about the research, programs, and progress.

FROM HIS SISTER, AKA MY AUNTIE SHERRE

I thought your dad was so cool growing up. We were seven years apart in age and grew up in the post-World War II Technicolor splendor of the new baby boomer middle class. We lived in a new San Fernando Valley suburban housing development that was only 20 minutes from Santa Monica beach.

Your dad had great taste in music as he brought home vinyl from the Doors, Jimi Hendrix, the Beach Boys, and Roy Orbison. He played those records on the family's new walnut console Magnavox stereo, our mom's pride and joy. He enjoyed science fiction TV shows like Chiller, Creature Features and The Twilight Zone.

I really enjoyed watching the shows with him, but sometimes he did stuff to scare me like throwing a wet washcloth. Sometimes the family would go to double-feature drive-ins on Saturday nights.

Your dad's lifetime friends came from the neighborhood we grew up in. They'd walk down the street to each other's houses to hang out or walk to the Matador bowling alley, or to the James Monroe High School to play tennis. They really liked to get together to play cards. Ted would buy bags and bags of junk food and set it out on the counter prior to the games, so everyone could have a good time.

The family liked to get together and play cards after big dinners.
We had great times playing 5-card stud, Knock, 7-card stud, and Texas
Hold 'Em. Your dad's grandmother lived in Venice, where he went
regularly to play poker, where he eventually learned to play a mean
game. Our parents liked to gamble, and they'd often "swing through
Vegas" on the way home.

Ted was close to his dad, and they enjoyed a special bond that
included quail and duck hunting and fishing in both fresh water
and deep sea. They'd clean the fish on the back porch, and he would
shake the silvery, toothy barracuda just to scare me. Our mom would
cornmeal-coat the fish and fry them up. Your dad always took the bones
out for me.

When your dad's father passed away in 1969 from a stroke caused
by nicotine and extreme caffeine habits, he was never the same. His
college deferment was not much better when he pulled a low number in
the draft that year, and he was only 21 when he enlisted in the army.
He served time in Korea, where he met your mom and later married.

Nearly two weeks had passed after my father's passing, and the last Sunday
of the February would be a full moon. Diane Klund, a dear friend whom I
coached to ride her first full century bike ride, organized a full-moon snow
show excursion for that Saturday evening. As usual I participated along with
many others from our NSET group. It was dark by 5 p.m., and we were on
our way up the path by 6 p.m. I remember how cold it was that winter and
how much snow we got in the mountains. That evening I couldn't see the
mountains from the valley, but when we got to elevation by Boreal snow
resort, the clouds were scattered and the moon was as bright as ever.

The Wailers were slated to perform that evening at the Grand Sierra
Resort, so I planned to meet Aaron Dehart at the venue around 9 p.m. when
I returned from the mountain. How I longed to see them perform "3 Little
Birds" by Bob Marley. In the first days of my dad's passing, I would play that

song, sing, and cry, "Don't worry; about a thing. Because every little thing. Gonna be alright." Well, they played it, and again I cried.

Within two weeks of my dad's passing, my soul grew wiser. I never felt so strongly about wanting to be a father and nurturing my own little one. My dad was a great man, and I know I wouldn't need to look far to find him.

I came to find great peace in knowing that my dad had passed before me. There would be nothing worse to face for my mom and dad than if I didn't make it through chemo. He knew that Ironman Canada was of utmost importance to me, and I had to find a way to get back to training. I trained only for a total of 88 miles in February. Not only did I have to make up for lost time but I'd have to regain the fitness that I lost. In essence I lost a month of training, and I had six months until Ironman Canada.

But just like riding a bike or being diagnosed with cancer, the only way you can keep from falling over is to keep moving forward.

February Training Mileage:
1.75 Swim, 59 Bike, 28 Run
TOTAL: 88.75

MARCH – A SHIFT IN PRIORITIES

Ryan Ress called during my crisis and wondered what happened to me. I apologized and informed him about my dad. There was a lot of work to do on my end for Spring Into Action 5k, particularly T-shirt sponsorship sales and getting the word out for our event.

My father's passing kept me away from work for two weeks. The owners were gracious enough to pay me for one of those weeks, and the second week came out of my PTO. Everyone at Access Pass & Design was cognizant and sensitive to what had happened, and no one asked questions about related events.

It was business as usual, and I realized the best thing I could do was to return to work and get back into a routine. The emotional toll, however, shifted my priorities, and I downshifted many of my business development initiatives from the new opportunities I harvested to just going through the motions.

Emotionally I was drained, physically I was weary, but mentally I was decisive. Instead of treating work life and Ironman training as equals and My Hometown Heroes second to that, Ironman training became my number one priority. My Hometown Heroes was second, and Access Pass & Design third. 2010 was my year—the only chance in my lifetime to celebrate ten years of brain cancer remission with an Ironman race, albeit my first one!

A true nonprofit organization has a classification called 501(c)(3) status. This means that the entity is tax exempt, and donations are tax deductible. You can only go so far without one, especially when it comes to asking corporations for financial support. Most of them want or need something to write off.

To acquire 501(c)(3) status, you must go through a lengthy application process and thoroughly complete a government-issued 1023 application. I delegated this task to one of my board members, who relied on a contact who never came through for us. My initial hope was to have the 1023 complete and mailed to the IRS by the end of March. I tried to complete the application myself, but between work obligations and my personal hardship, I simply tabled the process in May so I could stay mentally focused with Ironman training.

My momentum and enthusiasm to pursue hot business opportunities from LA and Baltimore came to a halt. All of the opportunities that I was so excited to pursue in Baltimore dissolved in the wake of losing my dad. However, sales were the best they had ever been for me in the first quarter of 2010, thanks to a few prosperous sponsorship activations from agency clients. And those sponsorship activations were a result of five years of relationships. It pay$ to stay in the game.

The afternoon following the Spring Into Action 5k, I flew to Chicago, where I met one of my coworkers, Stephen Person, who lived in Las Vegas. Stephen sold himself to Access Pass & Design after the ticketing company he had worked for went out of business due to the recession. Stephen was a good dude and brought new ways of thinking to Access.

The conference we attended was called International Events Group, better known as IEG. The IEG conference is an industry-leading event that brings people together for sponsorship consultation, measurement, and strategy.

IEG offered a six-hour preconference seminar called "Good for Business: Nonprofit Partnerships that Build Social and Financial Value." It was a $400 investment, which I paid for personally in order to attend and learn for the benefit of My Hometown Heroes. It really helped me understand the importance of partnerships, principles, and making the sponsor a relevant partner in the charity. Suddenly partnership opportunities became relevant for My Hometown Heroes with several of my current clients at Access. I was really excited for the potential, once I had time to establish my business foundation.

The networking opportunities and attendees who represented some of the top corporate brands were very approachable and open to new ideas. I walked away from IEG with an order from Australia's largest sports marketing agency, which was ready to ship by the time I returned to the office. More than anything, most of the people I met were excited to learn about My Hometown Heroes, my story, and my quest to finish Ironman Canada for my ten-year milestone.

ROAD TO IRONMAN CANADA

Between my father's passing in February and work travel, I lost a month of training and a significant level of fitness. All of the endurance running base that I built in training for the Las Vegas Marathon was depleted. I had ridden my road bike only once in a 30-day period and only ran 26 miles in four weeks. My mileage between swim, bike, and run in February totaled 89 miles, which was down nearly 25 miles from January. In March the total was

196. Within the first quarter I trained for a total of 400 miles, and I would like to have been at least 600.

Ironman Canada was less than five months away by the end of March. If I were to compete and finish within my goal time of less than 13 hours, I needed to focus with unwavering attention and dedication. That's all there was to it.

March Training Mileage:
3 Swim, 164 Bike, 29 Run
TOTAL: 196

APRIL - LAY OF THE LAND

Reno is surrounded by mountains and foothills. It's in a high-elevation desert at roughly 4,400 feet above sea level. The thinner air allows Reno athletes to build much greater lung capacity than those closer to sea level. I've seen the effects firsthand on cyclists from Florida, Texas, and Los Angeles when they rode AMBBR. They often comment about their struggles at the higher altitudes over 6,000 feet. That's one of the many perks of living at elevation, since most triathlons and marathons occur below 1,000 feet.

The climate between spring and summer can often fluctuate from cold, snowy winter conditions to blistering hot summer afternoons. I've been in Reno long enough to see snow in the valley in June and 90-degree temperatures the following week. The adverse weather conditions sometimes make it difficult for training rides. Sometimes high winds or wind-chill freezing temperatures will make a decision not to ride on a given day an easy one.

The Virginia foothills are on the south end of Reno where I live. The foothills intersect with highway 341, also known as Geiger Grade. It's a very windy road that climbs ten miles for a 2,300-foot elevation gain, peaking at 6,789 feet. The climb offers breathtaking views of the snow-covered Sierras and a great panorama of Reno and of Washoe Valley, which is nine miles to the south. I often imagine myself as a bird that's about to take flight on a fast downhill from the summit. Four miles beyond Geiger Grade's summit is the famous, old western mining town of Virginia City.

Further south of Reno, highway 395 will take you through Washoe Valley to Carson City, Nevada's state capital. For the most part Washoe Valley is flat but can get very windy in a very short amount of time. My dad drove through Washoe Valley every day for work. He'd often mention seeing diesel trucks and trailers that were tipped over due to the high winds. It's a scenic road, and many cyclists begin their routes at Bowers Mansion. The loop around Washoe Valley is approximately 21 miles.

Carson City has some very scenic side roads that *Team in Training* often utilized to avoid downtown traffic. These roads would eventually connect to highway 50, where you can turn right and drive to Spooner Summit and drop down into South Tahoe. However, if you were to bypass highway 50, highway 395 would lead you to Jacks Valley Road.

Jacks Valley Road takes you eight miles to a small, quaint town named Genoa, where cyclists often stop to rest or refuel on long training rides. There is plenty of shade and a sandwich shop that sees a lot of business over the summer. Twelve miles further south is Fredericksburg Road. Fredericksburg makes a great turnaround point for a 40-miler, out-and-back ride from Jacks Valley.

Just shy of one mile south along Fredricksburg Road, the California-Nevada border is distinctly marked. The road on the Nevada side is faded and light gray, whereas the pavement on the California side is black, smooth, and always seems fresh. With *Team in Training* we often continued south for the Diamond Valley loop. It was a group favorite, and if you ever drove or rode it, you'd know why.

Fredericksburg Road heads nearly five miles due south until it ends at Carson Pass Highway. The road T's off right and left, and either direction will loop back to where it began, if one's goal is to complete the Diamond Valley loop. Left will put you directly on Diamond Valley Road, and right will take you along the Carson River. Either direction is uphill, and I always preferred the Carson River route. It's the only river from South Reno on that particular route, and I always found it serene because there is seldom any traffic. It's nestled in a canyon, which blocks the wind while riding through.

The road stretches four miles and goes through Woodfords. There is a bait and tackle shop in Woodfords, where our group often stops to refill on fluids before proceeding to finish the Diamond Valley loop. An out-and-back from Jacks Valley to Diamond Valley is 60 miles. An out-and-back from Bowers Mansion to Diamond Valley is 85 miles.

Thirty-eight miles west of Reno along I-80 is Donner Lake, and just before you get to Donner, there is an exit to highway 89. Highway 89 will take you approximately 14 miles south, as you pass by two major Sierra ski resorts, Alpine Meadows and Squaw Valley. Squaw Valley was home of the 1960 Winter Olympics. At the end of the 14 miles is 64-Acres Park.

You can also take the highway 89 exit to get onto Donner Pass Road, which will take you past Donner Lake and to a 1,000-foot, four-mile climb to historic Donner Summit. Continuing just over four miles west of Donner Summit is the on-ramp to get back onto I-80, but there is a bridge that takes you over the highway and onto a side road that traverses I-80 called the Alan S. Hart Freeway. This freeway will take you on a fast, nine-mile downhill grade to Cisco Grove, where the road ends some 35 miles from 64-Acres Park. The 1,200-foot climb back up to the other side of Donner Summit was always a great endurance and strength builder at roughly 6,500 feet in altitude.

With the exception of the Chico Century and Indian Valley Century rides, those routes became my primary terrain for both preliminary and peak training months. I trained on all of these routes during my tenure with *Team in Training.*

TRAINING TIME

April was the first month of the year without any planned events or business travel. It was also my first opportunity of the year to get ingrained into a training routine. Tuesday evenings were my usual runs with NSET at 6 p.m.

with distances between eight and ten miles. Wednesday mornings I swam one mile before arriving at the office. Every Thursday evening I instructed my usual spinning class at Gold's Gym.

On the weekends I focused on longer miles for the run and the bike. I didn't necessarily start from scratch, but my mileage and fitness levels were only two thirds of what I wanted them to be. The Auburn Triathlon was less than two months away, and I had my last business trip ahead of me during the first week of May. I needed to rack up miles whenever I could, but it was a long winter and circumstances sometimes prevented workouts. The first weekend of April it snowed, so instead of cycling, I skied black diamonds at Mount Rose.

The second weekend, April 11, I rode what I like to call the Washoe-Geiger loop, which is exactly 56 miles and goes counterclockwise. It starts from South Reno heading south on highway 395 to Washoe Valley. From Washoe Valley the route takes you along the Franktown loop, down Combs Canyon, and continues south to an Arco gas station just shy of highway 50. From the Arco there is a bike lane that goes back north and intersects with highway 50, then goes five miles east on a gradual uphill to highway 341. From highway 341 it's eight miles to Virginia City, accompanied by 1,300 feet of elevation gain. Four miles north on a windy Geiger Grade will take you back up to the summit for a speedy ten miles of downhill back into Reno. On Sunday, April 11, I did my first brick workout on my Washoe-Geiger loop followed by a three-mile run.

The ride that took place on Sunday, April 18, was absolutely gorgeous with the snow-covered Sierras as our backdrop. Nicole Vaillant, who was training for her first Ironman triathlon and also a team member of NSET, also came along. She was training for Vineman Ironman course, which would take place a month before Ironman Canada. We would lean on each other frequently for moral support during our time of training. I led a 65-mile ride with NSET on the following weekend with a group of eight. It began at Jacks Valley Road and made its way to the Diamond Valley loop.

The majority of our group rode 40 miles, while Nicole, Brian Fruechtenicht (an NSET colleague), and I continued along for 65 miles.

Dave Fish set me straight on my training diet. I asked what he ate while training for an Ironman triathlon. His diet primarily consisted of steak, chicken, fruits and vegetables. He avoided pasta, breads, rice and other starch based products. I followed Dave's advice and had a big steak dinner, baked potato and salad on a Friday evening. My energy was longer sustained during my ride the following day, and ever since then I removed pasta, bagels and breads from my training diet. The quality of my workouts notably improved. You truly are what you eat.

The Chico Wildflower Century took place on April 25, where I had a chance to catch up with my cousin Jan Crane, Uncle Marvin's daughter. It was nice to see her along with her husband Bill, daughter Katie, and son Nick. I spent the night at their house, and we enjoyed a nice dinner together.

The official course map of the Chico Wildflower Century isn't 100 miles, and depending on whom you ask, the actual century course is between 93 and 95 miles. Over the years with *Team in Training*, I rode the metric century five times out of six, and I completed the full century once. The full century has a total elevation gain of 4,300 feet and begins with a base elevation of roughly 130 feet. There are three major hills along the course: Humboldt Road, Honey Run, and Table Mountain. Just over four miles into the ride, Humboldt Road is a short climb of three miles for 700 feet of climbing. Honey Run begins at roughly 240 feet and gains 1,500 feet of elevation over 12 miles. Table Mountain is a shorter climb with a steeper grade, which starts at 325 feet and climbs to 1,384 feet within eight miles of climbing.

Although the Chico Wildflower Century is rightfully known for the wildflowers that bloom along the course, the course's beauty wasn't as apparent to me as it was in 2010. The passing of my father and the ten-year remission milestone gave me a keener sense of appreciation. In years past, the ride had been more about helping others train for a century bike ride.

Table Mountain is the reason why the 100-mile bike ride is rightfully named the Chico Wildflower Century. It's a plateau where 200-foot-tall dark volcanic rock cliffs overlook a vast valley. The volcanic soil, marshy conditions, and natural irrigation to the valley below create the ideal conditions for its natural grand wildflower garden. The bloom is supposedly at its best in February and March, but April was quite spectacular, also. Blankets of yellow and violet canvassed much of the mountain, doused with spots of pink and orange. It was truly a sight to take pause and photograph.

At the beginning of the descent from Table Mountain, you're roughly 55 miles into the ride. Then there's a speedy downhill stretch prior to lunch. The remainder of the course is mostly flat and is surrounded by crops and orchards.

April Training Mileage:
4.5 Swim, 276 Bike, 70 Run
TOTAL: 350.5

MAY - BUILDING MY HOMETOWN HEROES

Since my attempt earlier in the spring to file for 501(c)3 nonprofit status had fizzled, I resorted to doing what I knew how to do best and created an online fund-raising page for My Hometown Heroes to coincide with my Ironman training.

The goal was simple: raise $10,000 for My Hometown Heroes to symbolize ten years of cancer remission. I got creative with my efforts and made donation levels to reflect various triathlon distances into currency:

Sprint = $25
Olympic = $50
Half Ironman = $70.30
Ironman = $140.60
Endurance = $250
Survivor = $500
Scholar = $1000

The fund-raising page was up by May 15, and I announced the platform through Facebook, Twitter, e-mail, personal letters to repeat donors, and clients.

Meanwhile I consulted with NSET's web developer, Jeff Moreland, who graciously donated his time to help set up a donation button on My Hometown Heroes website. Jeff replied, "Yep, I should be able to help you out. I don't mind helping you for free, but I can't commit to doing a lot for you. Your MHH website looks good so far. I can get started with an administer-level user login, password, and link to the admin page for the website. I'd probably need FTP access to the source files on the web server."

MORE TRAINING AND TRAVEL

May was a difficult training month, and day one was on a weekend. Saturday morning began with the Washoe-Geiger cycling loop followed by a one-mile swim in the pool. On Sunday I ran the Rock n' River Half Marathon and was on a plane to Chicago for the Event Marketing Summit by noon.

My workout regimen in Chicago was to get it whenever I could and concluded with two three-mile training runs. I restrained myself from getting too involved in late social networking activities, but I did have a few cocktails each night and perhaps stayed out a wee bit late on one night. Upon my return to Reno on Thursday afternoon, I was back in town early enough to instruct my 5:30 p.m. spinning class.

As expected, the training weekend was a flop as I took the conservative route to recover from my Chicago trip with a ten-mile run and a 35-mile bike ride. I understood my body's signs of fatigue and backed off when I felt I was on the brink. I was walking on a thin line and didn't want to compromise my immune system with only two weeks until the Auburn Half.

Open-water swims with NSET didn't take place until June. The water temperatures at Donner Lake and Lake Tahoe were simply too cold. The indoor swimming pool at Gold's Gym was the main reason I wanted to work there. On the weekends the gym allowed open swim times for families.

When kids are in the pool, there always seemed to be a higher propensity for bacteria, with coughing and sneezing.

On the first weekend of May, I swam one mile in somewhat murky water during family swim time. At first I thought the low visibility was due to the fact that the gym hadn't yet filtered the water. But when I swam on the third weekend of May, the water seemed even more cloudy than the previous session, and of course it was family swim time. I only swam a half-mile and left the pool feeling somewhat disgusted. My immune system consequently broke down, and I caught the flu with only eight days until the Auburn Half.

With antibiotics the virus cycled through my body in six days, which left me with two days until Auburn at 60 percent health at best. My goal was to finish in under six hours; but because of my setback with the flu, I reduced the goal to simply finishing the race as a means to log training miles. This was extremely discouraging. It was then I decided that I would never swim in a pool again during family swim time while training.

Dave Fish sent me an e-mail on May 21, the day I kicked the flu.

Hey Danny,

Good luck and kick ass in the half. My calf is still giving me trouble, so I won't be down there. Race like it's an Ironman at Ironman pace and get used to eating on the bike and get the nutrition thing nailed.

Have Fun.

Dave Fish

AUBURN TRIATHLON: THE WORLD'S TOUGHEST HALF - MAY 23

My college friend Brian Davis was from Auburn, California, and his family graciously welcomed me as their guest to spend the night, the evening before the race. Before dinner we drove to Rattlesnake Park, where the swim start began off the boat dock of Folsom Lake. The 1.2-mile swim would be two loops, followed by nearly seven miles of biking uphill with more than 900 feet of elevation climb.

The Auburn Triathlon allows athletes to place their running gear at T2, where the end of the first climb begins to level off. It was also this location where athletes claim bike rack position, which is exactly what I did, along with several other participants. Because of the late winter and temperamental weather, there was a high likelihood of rain that night. All gear was placed in plastic bags so that clothes would stay dry overnight. Bikes would be brought to T2 in the morning.

Following gear dropoff, Brian and his lovely wife, Mallory, treated me to dinner that evening along with their kids. We ate at an Italian restaurant. I slept soundly that evening on a pullout bed and woke to a drizzly and chilly Sunday morning. Brian prepared a light breakfast, and I was out the door by 5 a.m.

To get to the start from T2, athletes either rode down the hill to Rattlesnake Park or had family or friends drive them down to the start. Most rode down. The outside temperature was in the low 40s with a windchill factor that was near freezing. The lower elevation of Auburn compared to Reno often meant outside temperatures in the 50s or 60s in the morning at that time of year. The 6.5-mile downhill was torture on my hands because I didn't bring long-fingered gloves. My fingers and ears felt like icicles. In fact the air was so cold, Folsom Lake was covered in a layer of fog. The 64-degree water temperature nearly felt like a spa compared to the brisk outside air.

The race began at 6:30 a.m. for everyone under the age of 44. Women and other age groups would follow in three-minute intervals. The elite swimmers quickly distanced themselves from the masses. On the second-to-last turn of the second lap, the range of visibility was 20 feet at best, so I simply stayed in the middle of the pack, assuming they were heading in the right direction. It turned out they weren't, and we were about 25 yards from undercutting the final outer turn buoy. The course officials, in kayaks, indicated the final-turn buoy that we had to go around, which added several minutes to the swim.

My overall swim time could not have been good, but I didn't care to look back as I ran up the boat dock and around the bend to T1. I brought layers to accommodate the weather conditions but made my decision on what to wear based on watching those riding out. I decided to wear my cycling jersey and arm warmers for my upper body, which was enough to keep me warm on the uphills, but the downhills were still quite chilly. However, there was no turning back, and I would have to deal with the conditions for 56 miles.

When I began the bike leg, *Just get it done* was my attitude. The majority of the bike course was rolling hills with long, steep ascents and rapid down-hills. Nothing about the course was flat or easy.

It wasn't long before the course took its toll on my body, especially coming off of the flu. Riding uphill was usually my strongest discipline between cycling and running, but it was definitely my greatest handicap in this race. I had never gotten off my bike to push it up a steep hill, and I often gained most of my time on uphills during past races.

There is a 5.7-mile loop at the furthest point of the course that's called the Roller Coaster. Race directors caution athletes about it because, if you don't heed the signs to slow down, there is a high probability you'll launch off a ledge. They described this at the safety meeting the day before.

At the bottom of the loop is the Bear River, and the course actually flattens out for a mile or so. However, I needed to climb out of the ravine that I had gotten myself into from the Roller Coaster downhill. There was one section that got so steep on the uphill, I simply could not pedal further and unclipped from my bike to walk it up. At that point I began to contemplate if I would even finish the race. Mentally I had never been to this point of exhaustion and despair in any race, and I still had at least 20 miles to go on the bike course, the majority of which was uphill.

Three hours and 51 minutes later, I completed the grueling 56-mile bike course. The second I got off that bike, I said to myself, "Fuck this bullshit, I'm finishing this race." Needless to say, I was quite elated to be off that bike.

I've never quit a race because it was too hard. I certainly didn't quit when I had brain cancer, and I wasn't about to quit now. I had a full Ironman triathlon to complete in just over three months and two more half Iron distances before that. Mentally I had already finished the race, and it was only a matter of getting my body to follow suit. I finished the half marathon in 2 hours 7 minutes. Done! I was exhausted, but finishing this race was a huge shot of confidence for the next two 70.3s to follow. My finish time was 6 hours, 41 minutes.

The following week I drove to Quincy to meet with some friends to ride the 100 mile Indian Valley Century. I felt surprisingly great, considering the beating I took in Auburn.

May Training Mileage:
7.25 Swim, 349 Bike, 62.5 Run
TOTAL: 418.75

JUNE

Registration for Vineman 70.3 opens on November 1 every year. At that time in 2009 I hadn't fully formulated my training schedule and decided to wait. By the time I did decide to register on December 18, 2009, the race was sold out but had a waiting list of over 400 people. I was in the mid 400s, which seemed very high and somewhat uncertain.

Vineman was a critical race because of its timing in mid-July, which would be six weeks out from Ironman Canada and give me another opportunity to focus on any weaknesses. The waiting list still grew and was over 700 when I checked in January.

I contacted the registration administrator and asked what the likelihood was for people cancelling. She said, "Many people cancel, and even at your position on the waiting list, you'll have a good chance to make the cut. But

I can't guarantee anything." I checked the list weekly. Slowly but surely it began to condense, and before I knew it I was in the top 100.

On June 4 I received the following e-mail:

This e-mail is to inform you that you have been accepted off the waitlist for the 2010 Vineman Ironman 70.3. Please read the instructions below, and then follow the link to sign up for the race.

You will have seven days to complete your registration process. After that date you will no longer be considered for the event, and your name will be removed from the waitlist acceptance list.

The first thing I did was register for hotel accommodations at the same Travelodge where I stayed for the Vineman 70.3 in 2006. The hotel was in Santa Rosa, and it was a 17-mile drive to the race start. I registered for the Vineman 70.3 the very next day.

June 4 was also the day when Steve Oaks, Clarisse Mayer, and I began finalizing plans for the Boise 70.3; both were great friends from our days with *Team in Training*. Clarisse had friends in Boise who offered their home for us to stay in while we prepared for our race. I also had fraternity brothers in Boise whom I hadn't seen in over ten years, so it was a good opportunity to catch up with Chris Larose and Sean Coyle.

I exchanged e-mails and phone calls with Chris and Sean. Sean's initial reply was, "Good to hear from you! Yes, I should be around. My wife works 12-hour shifts Thursday through Saturday, so I'll have two kids in tow. Let me know your schedule and where you're staying, etc. BTW, I think part of the course goes right by my neighborhood. I can hand off a Coors Light if you need it. Ha ha."

Unfortunately Sean wasn't able to make dinner, since he got tied up with his kids and had to stay home. Chris, on the other hand, was one of my pledge brothers, and he was able to make it happen. In fact Chris met his lovely wife, Bobetta, while we were in college, so it was a great opportunity to catch up with the whole family.

Chris was from Vallejo, California, and was known for cooking up some mean barbeque while living in the Pike house. "Just let me know what you need, brother, and I'll hook it up."

"Anything packed with protein will do, as long as it's not fried. Steak, chicken, pork chops, and salad is all good stuff," I replied.

THE ROAD TO BOISE

Access Pass & Design had a sweetheart of an administrative assistant named Deb Ulp, who also managed the company's Facebook page. Deb also worked part time for a trial science psychologist named Dan Dugan, in hopes that she would be hired by him full time.

Deb always thought and spoke very highly of me and shared my cancer story with Dan. Dan was the lead advocate in the Reno area for the Livestrong Foundation, so there was great alignment. Dan's son, Chris, was also registered to compete in Boise 70.3.

Chris was 19 at the time and didn't have anyone to accompany him on the 425 miles between Reno and Boise. Steve, Clarisse, and I drove together in my Subaru Outback with two bike roof racks, and we loaded the third in the hatchback. Chris followed us in his dad's Suburban and stayed in a hotel he had booked earlier.

My last training ride before Boise was a 57 miler followed by a 3.5-mile running brick on Sunday, June 6. We left town on the morning of Thursday, June 10. About halfway to Boise we drove through a rainstorm, and I remember that the dark, gray clouds reminded me of the color of my Subaru Outback. I certainly hoped the storm wasn't a sign of what the weather might be like for the race. It was late afternoon by the time we arrived in Boise. Steve and Clarisse dropped me off at Chris Larose's house and then drove to Clarisse's friend's house, where we would stay for the next three nights.

Chris and Bobetta had three beautiful kids. It was great to hang out with the family and share memories of our days in college. Chris made food aplenty with barbequed pork chops and potatoes, while Bobetta made a wonderful garden salad. Chris was the same as I remembered him, very positive, witty, hardworking and family oriented. He always told great stories, which made him a great salesman. He was well versed in motor sports and was now an independent sales rep who traveled frequently to sell watercraft.

I traveled a lot for Access Pass & Design over the years, but not nearly as much as Chris. I admired all of the sacrifices he made to provide a wonderful life for his wife and three kids was glad we were able to share time together. Steve and Clarisse picked me up around 8:30 p.m., after they had dinner with their friends. Melissa was a good friend of Clarisse's, and we stayed at their place, along with her kids and her husband, Phil.

On Friday morning, I woke up and ran a few miles to perk up and awaken my muscles from the long drive. We enjoyed breakfast together and drove to pick up our race packets at Boise Centre around 11 a.m. The registration line was long, and it took us nearly two hours to finally check in and receive our timing chips and race bibs. We ate a light lunch and drove to Lucky Peak Reservoir, where we would check the water temperature and drive the bike course.

The late winter had a lingering effect in Boise, as it did in Reno and Auburn. The water temperature was reported at 53 degrees from the bottom of the dam, which meant a frigid 58 degrees on the surface for the swim. The bike course was pleasant at the start and began with about four miles of downhill along the Boise River, then up its first rolling hill.

Boise reminded me of Reno. It has many similar features, such as the high elevation desert climate, rolling foothills on the outside of town, and the Boise River running through the heart of downtown, similar to the Truckee River that runs through downtown Reno. If Sean Coyle and Chris LaRose enjoyed living in Reno it was clearly evident why they also enjoyed Boise.

Clarisse's friend Michelle, her husband, Phil, and their two kids were very hospitable. Phil played in a band. They also had a piano that Clarisse and I tinkered on. But the thing I remember the most about Michelle and Phil's home was the various life quotes they had hanging up on their walls.

The best one read:

> Thoughts become words
> Words become actions
> Actions become habits
> Habits become character
> Character is everything.

I took a picture of the piece and posted it on Facebook. A couple of friends commented:

> *Brian Kuykendall: Danny, I am proud of you for all you do, for all you have done, and for all you are about to accomplish! Keep up the hard work and dedication.*

> *Gene Kim: Did you make that, bro? I love this piece! Great way to start your day. Thanks for the positive message, my friend!*

JUNE 12 - BOISE 70.3

The Boise 70.3 is in a class of its own with a 2 p.m. start time; it's the only half Ironman–sanctioned event that begins in the afternoon. It's also near the summer solstice, so the sun doesn't set until after 9 p.m. which makes it a spectator friendly finish. Athletes finish in the heart of downtown Boise around dinnertime.

The late race start has its pros and cons. The obvious advantage is the opportunity to sleep in and prepare for the race without a great sense of urgency. Finishing in the heart of downtown when the city is getting warmed up for Saturday night activities is also something new to experience, as well as running along the river. Perhaps the two biggest downsides of the afternoon start time are a higher likelihood of wind during the swim and bike legs and adjusting to an unconventional fuel intake schedule.

T1 and T2 were in separate locations. T1 was at Lucky Peak Reservoir, while T2 was one block away from the finish line in the heart of downtown. This was also the first triathlon I would participate in that had wet suit strippers.

While Steve, Clarisse, and I enjoyed the luxury of a late start time, there was an agenda that needed to be followed. Running gear at T2 needed to be placed at the respective race number assignments on the bike racks between 10 a.m. and noon. T1 opened at noon for bike setup and body marking between noon and 1:45. The first swim wave began at 2 p.m.

Phil was going to pick us up at T2 and tow us to T1 along with our bikes. While we were waiting, I met a girl from Aspen named Catherine, or Cat, as she called herself. She was a ski instructor over the winter and a very strong and competitive cyclist over the summer. We exchanged numbers and have remained in contact ever since.

Phil dropped us off at Lucky Peak reservoir around noon, which gave us nearly two hours to set up before the race. By the time our transition area and body markings were finished, there was still over an hour before race time. Although I had snacks to hold me over, it was then I realized I probably hadn't consumed enough carbs or protein since breakfast—a couple of energy bars and that was about it. I hoped it wouldn't bite me in the ass during the race.

And so the race began in its respective waves of age groups. I was in the second wave of men between 30 and 34. We waded in the 58-degree water for about three minutes until the horn blew. One thing I did like about the swim was the yellow buoys on the way out. They were placed about 25 yards apart, which made it easy to keep a straight line. I had a natural tendency to swim slightly to the left.

My swim wasn't particularly great, but I was very much looking forward to the luxury of the time and energy to be saved when someone else would remove my wetsuit. But before a wetsuit can be stripped, the athlete must unzip the wetsuit from the back, peel off the Velcro from behind the neck, and pull out the arms. This can all be done while running to the designated area en route to the bike transition.

The procedure was simple. Sit on your butt, put your legs in the air, and the stripper will peel the remainder of the wetsuit from your body. At that point the stripper hands you your wetsuit while sunscreen girls lather you. Still, my T1 time was rather slow at 5:37.

Similar to my experience in Auburn, the bike leg was an absolute suffer-fest but with a completely different set of circumstances. Overall the bike course didn't come close in comparison to the hills in Auburn; but on this particular afternoon in Boise, headwinds and crosswinds gusted any where from 35 to 40+ miles per hour throughout the afternoon. The only part of the course where there was a tailwind was after the bike turnaround at mile 22, which was followed by nearly four miles of what seemed to be a 35- to 40-mile-per-hour tailwind, in which I easily sustained 40 miles per hour. That luxury was short-lived.

Around mile 40 there was a downhill section with a climb on the way out. But on the way back, it certainly was no downhill to be enjoyed. The headwinds were so gusty that I had to stand up and pedal to stay above ten miles per hour on a downhill that I would normally sustain 30 to 35 miles per hour without the wind.

By the time I got into town, I was mentally and physically tapped from the blistering winds and still had five miles to T2. It was an enduring flat five miles with slightly less headwinds, and I couldn't wait to be off the bike and onto the run.

Although not as windy or hilly on the five miles into town for T2, I was quite frazzled mentally. I longed to finish the bike leg and be on my way for the run. When I arrived at T2, I accidentally rolled my bike on the opposite side of the rack where my bike rack number assignment was located. So I had to roll my bike 20 feet down the aisle of racks and back up 20 feet to get to my assigned rack.

The run leg was actually very pleasant: two loops, flat, and sheltered from the wind, all on the Green Belt along the river. The run was my strongest leg, and I finished at the same pace I completed the Las Vegas Marathon, with a 8:24 average mile pace. My overall finish time was 5:52:08, and I placed 363 overall out of 1,401 participants.

By no stretch of the imagination was this an easy race. Due to the high winds on the bike, even the pros finished slower than in previous years. Craig Alexander, one of the world's best, finished with a time of 4:02:11 which was ten minutes slower than the year before.

Clarisse finished her first full Ironman Triathlon in 2005 in Coeur d'Alene, Idaho. In Boise, however, she only put in a small fraction of training effort for her 70.3. Because of the high winds during the bike portion, she converted her race to an aquabike. An aquabike is only the swim and bike portion of a triathlon.

Steve Oaks and Chris Dugan finished in over seven hours. Between Steve's bad hip and rigorous work travel schedule, he was limited on the amount of time he had to train. But he finished nonetheless, and I was there with Clarisse to greet and congratulate him when he finished. Steve was exhausted, and minutes after he finished the race he told us, "I just want to lay down."

When the medics saw Steve trying to relax off to the side, they immediately tended to him. "Are you going to be alright?" one asked.

"Yeah, I'll be fine," he replied.

The medic insisted that Steve come along with him to the aid tent to make sure all of his vital signs were functioning normally, and he supplemented Steve with fluids. By the time Steve was released from the tent, it was dark outside. Clarisse, Michelle, Phil, their daughter, and I waited in the front street courtyards where they served food and drinks.

I also waited for Chris at the finish line. I was nearly done with my race when he started his run leg. Chris's race was riddled with misfortune. A month prior to Boise he crashed during a bike race outside of town. He was unable to swim until race day and only rode twice since the crash.

Chris also experienced many firsts in Boise and none of them positive. It was his first half Iron distance race, which also began with his first flat tire. At one point his electrolyte bottle fell out of his cage, and he never bothered to retrieve it. "The wind almost made me quit on the bike course, and then during the run my blood pressure dropped drastically because I drank too much water and not enough electrolytes," he later commented.

The following morning, we all hobbled and moved around very slowly at Michelle and Phil's place. We ate breakfast with them for one last time and were on the road by 9 a.m. to pick up Chris at his hotel. Steve, Chris and I wore our Boise 70.3 shirts, and Clarisse took our picture as we stood side by side in front of my Subaru Outback with bikes on the roof. It was a great photo.

We drove back to Reno the way we came. About 30 miles out of Boise on the way to highway 95, we came to a cross street, and one of streets was called Chicken Dinner Road. We thought it was hilarious and wondered if there was a Fried Rice Drive nearby. We got out of the car to take pictures of each other in front of this hysterical road sign.

I rode back with Chris in his dad's SUV, while Clarisse drove my Outback. It wasn't until then that Chris and I really had a chance to talk and get to know each other. Chris was on University of Nevada's cycling team and raced competitively. Cycling was his number one passion.

Chris told me of a friend of his who recently finished her rounds of chemo and was attending BYU. Her name was Kristin Katich, and they became really good friends in high school through various leadership initiatives. We returned home around 6 p.m., and I was back at work the very next morning. Kristin would become My Hometown Heroes inaugural scholarship recipient in 2011.

Boise 70.3 – 5:52:08
Swim 41:19, Bike 3:10:53, Run 1:50:43
T1: 5:37, T2: 3:38
363 overall finish out of 1,401 participants

LIFE IN BETWEEN THE LINES

Living without my dad was hard. There were times in my dreams where he would visit, and I'd wake up crying in the middle of the night. I missed him so much. He never said a word, yet he was still my guardian angel, and I knew this when he was on this earth. Now he was watching me from above, just like he always did at my baseball games, tennis matches, bike rides, and graduations. He was always there.

Living without my dad brought on an entire new set of responsibilities, which revolved around taking care of my mom.

My dad took care of everything when it came managing finances, travel arrangements, record keeping, and staying in touch with family via e-mail. Now that he was gone, all those responsibilities fell to my mom, which meant they also fell on me.

There was never a necessity for my mom to learn anything on the computer. I patiently taught her the basics of e-mail, Billpay, and web browsing. She quickly got the hang of things after I made a few cheat sheets for her. And for the most part she became self-sustaining.

Between Ironman training, working full time, instructing a spinning class, and marketing My Hometown Heroes, I had more than enough to keep me busy. My mom had retired the previous Fall, and not only did she have to deal with the passing of my dad, she also had to figure out what to do with all of her newfound spare time.

She poured her energy into the church, and that kept her busy. She also juggled guitar lessons, piano lessons, and watercolor painting classes. But without a job her social life wasn't as involved as it once was. She had to learn how to deal with living alone.

We'd meet up for lunch or go out to dinner from time to time, and on May 16 the Broadway production of *The Wizard of Oz* came to Reno. I bought us balcony seats, and we both thoroughly enjoyed the show. When I was growing up, we'd always watch *The Wizard of Oz* movie together when it aired once per year on TV.

To help aid in the healing process, she decided she wanted to visit her family in South Korea and stay with her brother, my aunt and cousins. To be perfectly honest we needed a break from each other. I bought her plane tickets, and she flew to South Korea on June 16 and returned on July 5.

Without a doubt I was entering a critical phase in my Ironman training. After Boise 70.3, there were two and a half months remaining until Ironman Canada. Besides Dave Fish, a Keith Juhola (a fellow triathlete), and Nicole Vaillant, there was no one else to really train with at a similar capacity. A lot of the training was done on my own, which was somewhat intentional. I would be on my own for Ironman Canada, so it was time to get used to it.

June Training Mileage:
9.75 Swim, 304 Bike, 93.5 Run
TOTAL: 407.25

JULY

By the time July came around, I was deeply committed and entrenched in a weekly training ritual that went as follows:

Monday: Yoga for recovery
Tuesday: Swim laps from 1 to 1.25 miles in the morning, run 8 to 12 miles in the evening
Wednesday: Ride 25 to 30 miles after work
Thursday: Swim laps from 1 to 1.25 miles in the morning, teach spinning in the evening
Friday: Rest
Saturday: Ride from 70 to 100 miles, run 3 to 5 miles
Sunday: Open-water swim 1.5 miles, run 13 to 18 miles

Mid-June is generally when our training groups begin open-water swims in either Lake Tahoe or Donner Lake. However, the winter of 2010 was long and lingering. A few people from the NSET group planned the first open-water swim of the year at Donner Lake. This was two weeks following Boise 70.3. The long winter had its residual effects with the lake, as it was still much colder than what we were used to.

The swim workout goes just over .75 miles to what's known as Poop Rock. Poop Rock is a giant submerged boulder that barely surfaces from beneath and is the turn point on the out-and-back workout. When I reached the rock, I became dizzy, partly because of the elevation but primarily because the water was so cold. I vomited upon arrival.

As I swam back to shore, I could feel my body temperature drop. As I exited the water, I began to shiver, which was nothing entirely out of the ordinary at first. But the shivering continued uncontrollably. I was the only one from our group who didn't recover. My lips quivered and my teeth chattered for longer than I can ever remember. Shell, Keith Juhola's wife, commented that I was hypothermic and escorted me to the clubhouse, where they had a hot rinse shower.

I stood in the shower for nearly 15 minutes until my body stopped shaking and my fingers had feeling. After I regained my composure, I proceeded to ride my intended route to Cisco Grove and back for 40 miles.

Two weeks later, I received a group e-mail from RATS (Reno Area Triathletes) President Mike Ginsburg that read:

7/8

> We will swim this Sunday in Donner Lake. Those who braved the last swim faced some cold water. Good news: I just checked the temperature at the TD dock today, and it read 66 degrees, so it's definitely much warmer! Donner Lake Triathlon is a week from Sunday, so come out (or up for the Reno folks) for a practice in gorgeous Donner Lake.

I swam to Poop Rock and back with the group that Sunday, without any hypothermia issues.

I was very familiar with the Vineman 70.3 course, since I raced it in 2006. The swim is an out-and-back in the Russian River, where the water is so shallow at times that you can touch the bottom with your finger tips during the pullback of your swim stroke. There is a very mild head current on the first half and a tail current on the way back. The bike leg is a one-loop course with winding, rolling hills that peak with a sharp, 300-foot climb between miles 41 and 44.

What I remember the most about the run in 2006 was the extreme heat that lingered in the mid-90s. The course had a couple of mild, rolling hills on the out-and-back. I had gastrointestinal issues that year, and stopping twice for a rest stop during the run cost me anywhere from five to ten minutes. I finished with a chip time of 6:03:22 but beat my goal time of 6:15. I knew I had the capacity to do better.

Looking back at my 2006 cycling mileage, I logged 1,312 by the end of June. By the end of June 2010, I logged 1,208, but the difference in quality of miles between the two years was substantial. In 2006 I coached the TNT cycling group, so my rides were for the miles, not for speed. Although I competed in four triathlons in 2006, I only swam on race days, and my running mileage was maybe 15 miles per week at the very most in June and July.

By the end of June 2010, I had logged 31 miles in the water and 338 miles on the run since January. Plus I had two half Iron distance races under my belt. Overall I was faster in all three disciplines, more focused, and more determined.

July 2010 was not only my peak training month, it would be a breakthrough month on three separate levels. I gained, experienced, and capitalized on fitness levels that I didn't know my body was capable of achieving. It was the most fit I've ever been in my entire life, and it was truly amazing.

Between January and June I logged over 1,200 miles of saddle time. This consisted of two centuries, two 70.3 half Iron distance races, and a half marathon. On Saturday, July 3, I rode my third century distance of the year at 102 miles, followed by a three-mile run.

The following day was the Fourth of July, and I drove to Graeagle to compete in a sprint triathlon as a recovery workout that consisted of a half-mile swim, 15 cycling miles, and a three-mile run. It was a chore after the previous day's workout. On the run I began to feel strain on my left calf muscle, which persisted until Vineman 70.3 two weeks later. I had concerns.

Brian Kuykendall and his fiancé Denae had some family and friends over that evening to celebrate the Fourth. I partook in the festivities with a shot of tequila and a couple beers. I needed to let loose. Physically it was very relaxing. Mentally it worked wonders.

Aaron Hapgood is a good friend of mine from high school. We played varsity baseball and summer ball together, and we had similar tastes in music. When he found out I had cancer and survived chemo, there has always been a brotherhood bond since his dad passed away from cancer when he was in high school.

Aaron worked in the music business and was and still is a professional videographer. We'd occasionally see each other at concerts in my early days with Access, and he was a huge Dave Matthews fan. In fact the Dave Matthews Band was one of his clients whom he traveled with extensively every year to film.

I approached Aaron a few months before Vineman 70.3, shared my intentions with My Hometown Heroes, and asked if his schedule allowed him to interview me and film my race. He agreed to do it. We would meet in Sonoma to catch up at dinner the evening before the race.

JULY 18 - VINEMAN 70.3

The drive from the hotel in Santa Rosa to the race start in Guerneville was approximately 20 miles. Aaron and I were on the road by 5 a.m. on race morning and found a place to park in Guerneville by 6 a.m. The pro men's and women's swim was slated to begin at 6:30. All other age groups would start in six-minute intervals. The 33–34 age group was among the last of the waves and didn't begin until 8:22.

The morning air was cool with a blanket of fog resting on the warm Russian River—another sign of winter still trying to hang on. By the time I claimed my transition area, it was nearly 6:30.

Aaron and I had time to kill, so he interviewed me in front of the Russian River as the swim waves deployed. He hooked a mic on my shirt and started rolling film.

> Aaron: *Why are you here to race today?*
>
> Danny: *2010 is my tenth year of remission from brain cancer, and Vineman is my third half Iron distance of the year. I am training to compete in Ironman Canada to celebrate the ten-year milestone of being cancer free.*
>
> Aaron: *You're raising money for charity. Can you tell me a little bit about the cause?*
>
> Danny: *I started a scholarship fund for young cancer survivors as part or my ten-year celebration. It's called My Hometown Heroes, based off the inspiration and support from everyone who supported me as I endured three craniotomies and a year of chemo. They were my heroes.*
>
> Aaron: *What is it you wish to accomplish during today's race?*
>
> Danny: *Today is another opportunity to improve upon my previous half Iron distances this year, and I'd like to finish well under 5 hours, 45 minutes. But I think I'm capable of finishing faster, depending how good I feel on the bike.*

Aaron would try to post camera positions at various parts of the course, but the best opportunities for footage would be at my run start and run finish.

By the time 8:15 rolled around, I was on the beach waiting for the next swim wave to start so I could get in some warm-up strokes. When the start horn blasted for the next wave, I slowly began to walk into the water among the other athletes in my age group. We swam up the river for about 20 meters and back to get the blood flowing.

There were over 200 competitors people in my swim wave. Because my average rank in overall swim finish times is usually in the bottom third, I've learned it's best for me to start from the back and work my way into the line from the outside in. Every time I've tried starting in the front during any triathlon, I always find myself in a dangerous position of flying elbows, legs, and arms. It's never pleasant to get hit in the face by someone's foot or hand in the water.

There are, however, no age group starts in a full Ironman Triathlon. It's every person for himself or herself, and the clock will continue to tick no matter when you decide to enter the water. So, I needed to put myself into this hostile scenario, since Ironman Canada would be much the same. I made a race day decision at Vineman 70.3 to start my swim at the very front of the pack, in the middle.

I was overtaken in a matter of seconds when my age group began. It was very tight quarters, and I found myself quickly falling behind the pack. It seemed like more than ten minutes until I was finally able to get into my usual sub-40-minute 1.2-mile swim groove.

Because I was in the last wave of the day, the bike racks were almost completely empty when I emerged from the water. The majority of the competitors were well on their way along the bike course. And just like Vineman 70.3 in 2006, I struggled to make a decent transition time. The ground was covered with rocks and gravel, which caused me to walk slowly. By the time I was on my bike, however, I felt fast and efficient.

The total number of registered male participants was 1,261 among all age groups. To give you an idea of the competitive field, I finished 1,041 on the swim and 756 on the bike. The results website didn't offer rankings on the run, but I improved my times immensely on all three disciplines from my 2006 Vineman 70.3. With two marathons under my belt since 2007 and the Ironman fire within me, I began to understand what it was like to be Iron fit, a term used when Ironman athletes are entering the peak training zone.

Since 2006 my Vineman 70.3 swim time had improved by three minutes, my bike improved by eight minutes, and the most significant improvement was my run, which was nearly 14 minutes faster. My overall time improved by nearly a half hour, and I was pretty darn proud of that. Here are the stat comparisons:

2006 Vineman 70.3– 6:03:22
Swim 42.43, Bike 3:05.41, Run 2:04:35
T1: 5:11, T2: 5:10
819 Overall Rank of 1,536

2010 Vineman 70.3 – 5:35:53
Swim 39:15, Bike 2:56.01, Run 1:51:03
T1: 5:40, T2: 3:53
540 Overall Rank of 1,874

A LESSON

Dave Fish taught me a few valuable lessons over the years. I have him to thank for making me a better swimmer by indicating I was kicking way too much during our training swims in 2005. He inspired me to change my diet from carbs to protein while training for Ironman Canada. It made a huge difference in my overall sustained energy. He even influenced my travel logistics, from bike transport to travel arrangements to Canada. Flying into Spokane and renting a car to drive up to Penticton was clearly a better choice and shorter distance than flying into Seattle.

But the most valuable lesson I learned from Dave came the weekend following Vineman 70.3. That following Saturday I rode the typical Washoe–Geiger loop for 70 miles and felt incredibly good. On Sunday I joined Dave and some other local Reno triathletes for a 1.5-mile swim at Donner Lake followed by two run loops around the lake.

I arrived late. By the time I was finished with my swim workout, Dave and Nancy had begun their two laps, while I returned to the car to change into my running gear. I caught up to them within the first two miles and maintained my pace.

Overall my body felt strong until I got to mile nine on the second lap. I bonked and ended up walking much of the remainder of the course. Dave and Nancy came back around to pass me with just under a mile remaining. When I finished the workout and met Dave and Nancy in the parking lot, he asked, "What pace do you want to run your Ironman?"

"Ideally I'd like to maintain around an 8:30 mile pace," I replied.

Dave answered, "You may want to rethink that and start your run pace around 10:30 per mile. Then as you progress, you can pick up the pace if your body is feeling up to it. Run the race between 10 and 10:30 and try to continue at the same pace for about fifteen to sixteen miles. If you're feeling up to it, pick up the pace. You'll know how hard to push yourself from that point forward." I took Dave's advice to heart.

THE INTERVIEW

My schedule after Vineman 70.3 became somewhat hectic. A friend of mine helped arrange an interview with News Channel 2 to share my story, my Ironman pursuit, and My Hometown Heroes. The interview and filming took place in my office at Access Pass & Design with Wendy Damonte, a fantastic local news anchor. The interview was on the Wednesday after Vineman, and it broadcast the following Tuesday on her "Heatlh Watch" segment at 5:30.

Wendy: *Sure, Danny Heinsohn has your typical aches and pains from being an endurance athlete. You can see his leg wrapped for support during his training run. But there are other signs on his body of a time when pain was much deeper, much more scary.*

Danny: *I was diagnosed with a brain tumor in May of 1999, the day after I graduated college.*

Wendy: *He was just 23 years old, leaving to backpack across Europe. But his diagnosis changed that and his life. Friends and family surrounded him during three brain surgeries when doctors removed a tumor the size of a racquetball followed by a year of chemotherapy.*

Danny: *That was one of the valuable things I took away from this is that being there can make all the difference in the world. That gave me strength. And I fought. My whole reason for fighting was because of them. I didn't want to let them down.*

Wendy: *On his tenth-year anniversary of being in remission, he launched his own foundation, My Hometown Heroes, named in honor of those who helped him through his ordeal. The goal is to raise money for kids fighting cancer.*

Danny: *So I am training for Ironman Canada as my initial campaign to promote my organization.*

Wendy: *The Ironman consists of 2.4 miles of swimming, 112 miles on the bike, and a marathon. Danny has never competed in an Ironman event, but he has endured a similar hardship.*

Danny: *There are a lot of parallels with the Ironman and going through cancer. It takes a lot of will, it takes a lot of determination, and it takes a lot of support from friends and family.*

Wendy: *And so he continues down another long road—this time to fight for the youngest victims of cancer. The kids will walk in his shoes of chemotherapy in hopes of one day going to college on scholarship money raised from these shoes.*

BODY MAINTENANCE

I began making monthly visits with my chiropractor and my massage therapist once every few weeks. Dr. Day had been my chiropractor for over a year and worked wonders. I always felt centered and clear-headed after his adjustments.

My massage therapist, Diane Heluva, was magical as well. My first massage of the year was in April, and I decided to try a hot stone massage. I was hooked and would continue with hot stone massages for every session. She knew how to dig into all of my sore spots and make me squirm. We always seemed to get a good laugh every time I was in pain. She made me hurt so good.

Dr. Day and Diane were a part of my Ironman team and were always supportive and inquisitive of my training efforts. They were vital components to my training success.

THE WEDDING

Brian Kuykendall and Denae were slated to be married on Saturday, July 31. I missed Brian's bachelor party in May because of the Auburn Triathlon but was committed to attend the wedding. Gene Kim, Aaron DeHart, Dave White, Andy Dennis, Brian's brother Kenny, and I would all be in the wedding.

Brian's wedding was five weeks before Ironman Canada, and I had to modify my weekly training schedule since I couldn't train on the day of the wedding. Based on several articles I had read and on input from Dave Fish and Scott Robertson, three weeks is the common consensus for tapering before an Ironman. I was in somewhat of a pickle and decided to flip-flop my training routine. My long ride would take place on Sunday instead of Saturday, and I took Friday off of work to run 20 miles. There would be no open-water swim that weekend.

The wedding rehearsal was on Friday afternoon, so I had to be punctual with my training miles to give myself enough time to make it to the rehearsal in Tahoe. Towards the end of July the high temperatures were flirting with 100 degrees. I was exhausted after my training run on Friday and shortened the intended distance from 20 miles to 18 miles. Little did I know that that would be the longest training run before Ironman Canada.

After the wedding rehearsal, up in Tahoe, we all went out for pizza and beer. I limited myself to half a beer. On the morning of the wedding,

Brian gave all of his groomsmen flasks of Crown Royal with our nicknames engraved on them. On several occasions throughout the day, we raised our flasks to Brian and Denae and delivered speeches at the reception. My departure from the wedding was around 3 p.m., as I said my goodbyes and drove back to Reno.

Nicole Vaillant's Ironman was the same day as Brian and Denae's wedding. The Vineman Iron Distance course did not have an online athlete tracker, so a couple of Nicole's friends who attended the event posted updates on Facebook. I monitored and cheered her on through social media. She went on to finish with a respectable time of 13 hours and few seconds.

Meanwhile, the little amount of alcohol I consumed at the wedding threw my metabolism into a tailspin. My mind raced all night and I barely got any sleep for a time I needed it most. My plan was to ride 100 miles the following morning.

July Training Mileage:
12.75 Swim, 417 Bike, 97.5 Run
TOTAL: 527.25

AUGUST

August 1 was the day after Brian and Denae's wedding. I proceeded to follow through with my training intentions and rode from South Reno through Washoe Valley, Carson City, and Jacks Valley until I was within a couple miles of the California border. I then turned around to go back up the way I came for over 25 miles and finish the loop that included the ascent to Virginia City. I rode a total of 102 miles that day, which ended with temperatures in the high 90s. Overall I felt strong throughout the entire ride.

Depending whom you ask, the lifespan of a road bike tire can be anywhere from 1,000 to 2,500 miles. Of course the quality of the tire and the brand have something to do with that. I began my second set of tires on my specialized Roubeux bike in 2009. By August 2010 I was over 1,500 miles.

I wasn't entirely faithful in checking the wear on my tires and planned to purchase a new set before Ironman Canada. But intentions are no good if you keep putting them off.

On the second weekend of August, I was slated for a 70-mile moderate training ride. My ignorance got the best of me that day on the Washoe-Geiger loop. As I pulled through the switchbacks on the truck route to Virginia City, my front tire fired off like a 22-caliber bullet. I worried that the back tire might follow suit.

There was a significant gash on the surface where the tire blew. I had a spare tube and two CO2 canisters, but what was the point if the tire couldn't hold the pressure? I wasn't in a favorable location, being ten miles away from any city limits or modern conveniences. I decided to play MacGyver, walked myself and my bike to a large bush for shade, and got to work.

To fix the gaping hole, I placed two self-adhesive patches inside the tire to cover it. I pulled out the blown tube, cut out a 1-inch-by-3-inch rectangle, and folded it over three times. I lined the inside tire with the new tube and held the 3-fold in place with my index finger until it was snug and beaded inside the tire. It was a leap of faith and I only had one chance to get it right. The wait for anyone to pick me up would be anywhere from one and three hours, and I'd lose my training mileage for the day. It wouldn't be long until the sun was directly overhead and my fluids completely depleted. I couldn't afford to wait.

Fortunately the fix held the entire way back, including the 2,200-foot descent from Geiger into South Reno. I posted a picture on my Facebook page; the tire looked like bent rebar because of the uneven distribution of air pressure.

Somewhere between Brian's wedding and the 70-mile flat tire incident, I acquired a gum infection. I most certainly believe that the stress my body went through that last weekend of July was too much to fight off any sort of infection. With Ironman Canada four weeks out, I couldn't afford to get sick—not after all the miles, hard training, and invested emotions.

My cortisol levels must have been going through the roof after those shots of Crown Royal at the wedding followed by that 102-mile ride. It was like reliving the sleepless nights of going through chemo when my body couldn't keep up with how much it needed to metabolize (nor could my racing thoughts). Every workout in that two-week period was laborious and exhausting. I was forced to take two to three days off each week.

As for my lack of energy, it didn't dawn on me until I stepped on a scale two and a half weeks before Ironman Canada. My average weight is between 159 and 162, even while training. I was all the way down to 151 when I weighed myself at the gym with only two and a half weeks until Ironman Canada. My mental acuity and sleep deprivation reduced me to think, "At this point, I just hope to finish."

Somewhere among those long sleepless nights, I lost track of my protein intake and overall nutrition consumption. I scrambled to get back on a hearty diet and ate larger portions more constantly: steak, chicken, eggs, fresh fruit and vegetables, dairy, and even a few pastries. As I gained my weight back, I gained more energy.

The Saturday before I left for Canada, I rode 41 miles from Donner Lake to Cisco Grove and back, followed by a run lap around the lake. I felt like I was back on track with my Ironman training yet cautious not to push as hard as I did in some of the weeks in July. I was definitely walking the thin line that separated me from the proverbial wall and breakthrough fitness.

THE FINISHING TOUCHES

My last workout with NSET was on Tuesday night, August 17, a six-mile run. My running peers only saw me on Tuesday evenings, since my Saturday runs were replaced with long cycling miles. Nicole ran that day, and so did Dave Fish and Nancy.

Dave sent me a link from slowtwitch.com earlier that day from a guy who blogged about race preparation for Ironman Canada. He goes by the alias of jonnyo, and he had a lot of great insights and common-sense reminders: stick with your training plan, don't do anything out of the ordinary, stick with your regular eating habits, learn to relax, pace yourself, and suck it up if it gets tough.

Meanwhile Dan Dugan allowed me to borrow his bike transport case. With our common interests in fighting cancer, his affiliation with Livestrong, and his son Chris leading me to an introduction to my first scholarship recipient, we had a good thing going.

Chris Dugan's friend, Kristen Katich, and I finally connected at this time as well. We spoke briefly on the phone to share our abbreviated versions of our cancer stories, and then we exchanged a couple of e-mails. I asked if she could send me a one-page testimonial of her journey and sent her my essay "Regarding Hope."

8/18/10

Kristin –

Thank you very much for sending this. It shares a lot of the same types of references as the essay I completed during my third month of chemo. I'd like to share it with you. Please find attached. Let me forewarn you that it's 14 pages long, single-spaced, so you may want to block out some time :)

8/18/10

Danny –

I'll be sure to tackle that today. I can't wait to read it. I was treated for 2.5 years (828 days) but still have appointments every month and get hospitalized every now and then for complications. I am going into nursing. After all the time I spent in the hospital, I'd like to go back and be on the other side and empathize with my patients. I have a passion for art, but I don't plan on pursuing that for a career.

The rental car and flights for my mom and I were booked from Thursday,

August 26, through Tuesday, August 31. Thursday was a travel day. Our flight would depart from Reno at 7:55 a.m. and arrive in Spokane at 10:20 a.m. We'd pick up our rental car and drive to Penticton, 227 miles away, roughly five hours of driving. The rest of the trip went as follows:

Friday – Mild workout to make sure gear is intact

Saturday – Rest, relaxation, and mental preparation

Sunday – Ironman Canada

Monday – Sleep, hobble, massage, relish the accomplishment

Tuesday – Drive to Spokane, return to Reno

I notified my credit card company that I would be out of the country, so there would be a lift on international transactions during travel days. I made a checklist of everything I needed to bring. Frank at Access activated the roaming charges on my phone so I could call, e-mail, and post updates on Facebook.

On Tuesday, August 24, I saw Diane Heluva for one last one-hour hot stone massage. And on Wednesday Dr. Day made one last adjustment. Both of them were excited to hear all about it when I returned. Neither had ever worked on an Ironman triathlete, let alone a brain cancer survivor. My body was bouncing back to racing form, and for the first time since my nutrition tailspin, I began to feel ready.

GO TIME - THURSDAY, AUGUST 26, 2010

Everything was already pre-scheduled when we arrived in Spokane. The first thing we did was pick up the rental car with a trunk large enough to fit the bike case I borrowed from Dan Dugan. It was a Toyota RAV4. The next item of business was to eat after the 3.5-hour flight. We had a layover in Boise.

My hope was to be on the road to Penticton by noon after lunch in Spokane. We ate at a Mexican restaurant called The Azteca, where I topped off my phone battery since I forgot to bring my car phone charger. Not only did I forget to bring my charger, I also forgot to bring CDs for the road. My mom brought a few of her favorites, which included *Michael Jackson's Greatest Hits, Andrea Bocelli, Phantom of the Opera,* and *The Lion King.*

After about two hours my mom took the wheel, and we listened to the Michael Jackson and Lion King albums. I regained the wheel before crossing the border and we moved at a snail's pace through customs.

As we drove up highway 97, we passed Osoyoos, which was the turn point heading north on the Ironman Canada bike course. We continued driving northbound through the wine capital of Canada known as Oliver. We then drove past Lake Vaseux and Skaha Lake, and then finally into Penticton.

It was nearly 6 p.m by the time we arrived in Penticton. After checking into the Carmi Inn, I decided to jog lightly for a few miles to awaken my limbs after the long drive. Reno is roughly 4,400 feet above sea level where Penticton is only 1,263. I could definitely breathe easier and had the propensity to keep going. I had to restrain myself to four miles and return to the room so my mom and I could find a place to eat dinner.

We soon walked to a nearby Safeway to stock up on groceries and supplies for the long weekend. We bought all the regular fixings for a protein-packed omelet which included eggs, egg beaters, mushrooms, green onions, ham, and tomatoes.

The Carmi Inn had a kitchen and two separate bedrooms. Later that evening my mom was in her room getting familiar with The Jimmy Fallon Show on NBC, while I was reading about Penticton in my room. It was the first time she heard Jimmy Fallon, and she thought he was hilarious.

Meanwhile I was receiving plenty of encouragement from back home via Facebook with comments like:

Jud Domenici: *Tear it up, brother. I'm proud of you, and it's a pleasure calling you a friend!*

Denae Mezera-Kuykendall: *Danny . . . Good luck on your unforgettable adventure! We will be thinking about you and will be ready to celebrate with you when you return :)*

Katie Grever-Wendling: *Danny, my friend, today you're on your way to Canada. We are proud and will be tracking your race. I think you are right where you need to be. See you when you get home . . . PARTY!!!*

Amin Dan Haq: *BROTHA!!!!!! I can't tell you how proud I am to know such an incredible man. You're an example and motivation! Thank you for taking the time to keep us all up to date in little ways as you've made this journey from cancer to preparing for the Ironman in Canada. God Speed my brother. You are in such good hands.*

FRIDAY, AUGUST 27, 2010

Mom cooked up her famous omelet for breakfast, accompanied with toast and strawberries that she picked up the night before.

Compared to August 2009, Penticton was significantly cooler in 2010. It was cloudy. In fact rain was forecast for race day. My mom didn't bring a jacket or a good pair of running shoes, so we stopped by Wal-Mart. I picked up a ten-dollar gray hoody, and she purchased a purple jacket with a hood for $25, along with a generic brand of walking shoes.

My plan that morning was to swim one kilometer in Lake Okanagan, where Ironman Canada would start, followed by a 25-mile bike ride along the course. There are three legs to the swim. The first leg goes out 1,600 meters, turns right, then goes another 450 meters, and then it's 1,750 meters back to shore.

My mom took pictures of me in my wetsuit before I began the workout. For some reason I thought the initial leg was only 800 meters, but it was twice the distance. I felt so good on the swim that I went out nearly 1,000 meters, which meant I had to swim back the same distance—not exactly what I had in mind but again, I felt great.

We soon returned to the hotel, where I strapped on my bike shoes and helmet and went out for a 24-mile out-and-back along Skaha Lake. I felt strong on the ride and even incorporated a couple of sprint intervals. I felt like jumping out of my own skin I was so excited!

Following the workout we walked to packet pick-up for my bib number, timing chip, helmet and bike stickers, and special needs bags. My mom reminded me that I should schedule a massage the day after the race, which I did. My work was done for the day and the next. Saturday was a 100 percent day of rest.

RACE EVE - SATURDAY, AUGUST 28, 2010

Since the beginning of the year, I logged 2,511 miles of training between the three disciplines. That's 54 miles of swimming, 1,967 miles of riding, and 490 miles of marathon training in eight months.

My two-week nutrition setback that began after the first week of August left me with doubts about finishing within my goal of under 13 hours. At best I felt 80 percent of where I hoped to be on race eve. My goal splits were to finish the swim within an hour and a half, followed by seven hours on the bike, then complete the run within four and a half hours. I felt I had enough cushion to keep me close to a sub-13-hour Ironman finish, including transition times.

My race strategy was simple yet tactical: be well rested on race morning and never let myself go hungry. There was no more preparation left to do but remind myself of the little things.

One of the accommodating features about the Ironman Canada swim course is it's one of the longest shoreline starts in the Ironman series. Of course the fastest swimmers would start at the front on the right-hand side of the shore, while other tactical swimmers like myself would likely start midway on the shoreline and work into the line from left to right. I hoped to take advantage of the current created by the other swimmers.

The bike was still my strongest discipline. If I felt strong on the bike, then I would have a great marathon start. For the run I would follow Dave Fish's strategy of a sub-ten-minute-mile pace; and with 10 miles or so to go, if I was feeling good, then pick up the pace. At the end of the race, I wanted to finish strong.

During my peak months of training, I never went the full distance for any given discipline. My longest distances in separate workouts were a two-mile swim, a 102-mile bike, and an 18-mile run. I relied on my fitness base and mental capacity to complete each full distance throughout the race.

The pasta feed that evening took place at the Penticton Trade & Convention Center, where my mom and I met with Michelle and Brian. Jesse Viner called and left a voice mail just before I went to bed after 10 p.m. It was somewhat unexpected, but I was excited for the call. I forgot he mentioned he would be at a Green Day concert with his fiancé, Larissa, on the eve of the race. All I heard was distorted background noise and front man Billy Armstrong singing, "It's something unpredictable, but in the end it's right, I hope you have the time of your life."

I was moved to tears, played it once again, and sent him a text, "I love you, brother." I was sound asleep minutes later with the alarm set to go off at 4:30 a.m.

IRONMAN CANADA – SUNDAY, AUGUST 29, 2010

For nearly six hours I slept soundly and was wide awake before my alarm had a chance to summon me. I thought to myself, "This is it!" and listened to Jesse's voicemail one last time. I remained in bed to go over my mental checklist for the day's big event and reminded myself of a few things:

- Pace yourself.
- Never let yourself grow hungry or thirsty.
- Enjoy the day.

As planned that morning, my mom made an omelet, toast, and cut up fresh fruit—the same portion intake I would consume before a long training ride. I left the table to relieve myself in a big way during breakfast time. We loaded my bike and tri-gear into the rental car and made sure we both had what we needed for the day. We left the Carmi Inn and drove to the neighborhood where I planned to park, and we easily found a spot that was about 12 blocks away from the transition area. It was still dark at that hour with the faint glow of dawn along the eastern horizon.

There were several athletes marching toward the transition area with their families and friends. By the time we reached the entrance, there were hundreds of athletes already inside with their bikes already racked.

My bike rack location was fairly open, and I didn't have to squeeze between anyone to set up my transition area. I was comfortable that I arrived without feeling rushed and was able to lay out my gear in a calm state of mind.

It wasn't until 20 minutes before the race start that I began to put on my wetsuit. I took one last iPhone picture of the crowd of participants as they lined up along the shore of the swim start and posted it with a caption that read, "T-minus 19 minutes." I turned off my phone, packed it in my transition bag, and began the march to the swim start along with an army of 3,000 other participants from around the world.

In just minutes I would be living my wildest dream. Who would've thought that after being diagnosed with brain cancer and undergoing three craniotomies that I would eventually become an Ironman?

With less than a minute to go, Steve King the famous Ironman Canada announcer, made the following statements with less than a minute to start time, "We hope it's the greatest of days, we hope you have the time of your life". Music began to play. "20 seconds to start time so let's start counting down. 15 seconds away, join me in the countdown if you would. *10, 9, 8, 7, 6, 5, 4, 3, 2, 1.*"

I walked forward for one minute until I got horizontal in the water, and when I began my stroke, I thought to myself, *It's on!* The environment wasn't unfamiliar, but the excitement was unlike any other triathlon I had ever participated in. I was competing in an Ironman and all of a sudden I was in motion on the longest swim of my life. I steered clear of heavy swim congestion and maintained my stroke on the first mile out until the first turn, which was marked by a mini party yacht.

The first right-hand turn was a relief, and the stretch was short until the second turn. From there it was straight ahead for nearly 1.2 miles until I was out of the water. From that point in the lake, I couldn't even see the transition arch and just pressed forward while siting those around me. 2.4 miles was a long swim, and I was relieved to set foot on the ground. I slowly jogged to T1 and looked forward to the wet suit strippers.

By the time I was on the saddle, I was nearly five minutes ahead of my intended goal time which was to be out of the bike transition area within an hour and thirty minutes. I was elated to be on Main Street, the first stretch on the bike leg that is southbound and on the way out of Penticton. The crowd cheers along Main Street created a seismic wave of emotions that crashed into me. Tears of joy began to stream down my face; a polar opposite contrast from when I embraced my mom and dad when we first learned of my brain tumor in May of 1999.

The lay of the land was how I remembered it from the year before, with the exception of McLean Creek Road, which was approximately ten miles out of Penticton. I regained large amounts of time as I passed what seemed to be hundreds from the start, past Lake Skaha, up McLean Road and along Vasseux Lake.

A second wave of emotion crashed over me along Vasseux Lake. I felt a strong presence of my dad, and I knew he was right there next to me. No matter what came about during the day, he would be there for me, as he always was through thick and thin.

The weight of those moments took me out of the present for a short amount of time, and the next thing I knew, riders were passing me as if the emotions had somewhat slowed me down. During the next 10 miles I experienced my first and, thankfully, only moment of doubt. I still had 80 miles to go on the bike and hoped to pull out of my mental funk.

Then at one point around mile 35, I was about to pass a woman who stood up on her pedals coming down a hill. It appeared as if she had a carbonated energy drink that was erupting from her water bottle. As I pulled alongside and ahead of her, I realized she was urinating. It was gross yet somewhat amusing. I've heard of athletes urinating on the bike or run, but this was the first time I had ever seen it, so there was somewhat of a shock factor. Throughout the bike course I found that this wasn't so uncommon, as I noticed a few others relieving themselves along the way. I guess if you're trying to achieve a personal best or qualify for Kona, some will do whatever it takes.

I had to do the same at approximately mile 40, but I stopped and waited in line at a Porta-Potty. I waited nearly ten minutes until it was my turn. I factored a bathroom break or two in my race strategy and hoped this was the only time, which, thankfully, it was. It was a relief and I felt lighter when I got back on the saddle. From that point forward I was strong and focused for the duration of the ride.

Once we rode through Oliver, we were close to Richter Pass, the first of two passes on the course. And like training at Cisco Grove or Geiger Grade, I applied the same intensity. In fact I passed several riders, and nobody passed me up that hill. I felt amazing, and from that point forward very few people passed me on the bike leg for remaining 60+ miles.

After the epic descent from Richter, several athlete supporters in their cars were parked or driving to the next area of interest to cheer on loved ones. I would say that around mile 60, my mom and Michelle's family would pass me with cheers of support. I was absolutely ecstatic to see them, and we chatted briefly as they drove beside me. Within the next hour or so, I found myself at the out-and-back special needs pickup point, where I grabbed a zip-lock bag of Doritos, anti-seizure medication, and Advil. The Doritos were great, as they help replenish the salt content in my body.

While 2009 had been a fire season, there was a high chance of rain during the 2010 race. It was cloudy all day, and it only seemed like a matter of time before we would get wet. About ten miles after the special needs bag pickup, it began to rain and the wind-chill was brisk. I was drenched and had not yet begun the long ascent up Yellow Lake pass.

The crowds of fans and supporters were out in full force, just like they were in 2009. Traffic was gridlocked across the entire span of Yellow Lake. People were out of their cars and alongside the rode the entire way up. They didn't seem to mind the elements, and they cheered for everyone as they climbed that hill.

"Come on, you're almost there!"

"You're doing great!"

"The top is just ahead, and it's all downhill back into town!"

Those were the words I longed to hear all day. I was drenched, and I had a few up and down moments, but I was thoroughly elated upon reaching the top of Yellow Lake. It was downhill from there and then flat on the way back into Penticton. Aid stations along the bike course were approximately ten miles apart from each other, and by the time I reached the top of Yellow Lake, I had consumed three bananas, a bag of Doritos, a couple of Power Bars, five gels, and five bottles of hydration fluid.

I was soaked by the time I entered the transition area, but thankfully my T2 bag was full of dry clothes. It was pleasant to have volunteers rack the athletes' bikes upon entering T2 and hand off transition bags.

My saddle time on the bike was just over six hours and nearly an hour faster than my goal time of seven hours. That was uplifting. I was relieved to be off the saddle and in a chair to prepare for the run in the transition tent. The volunteers were extremely helpful and willing to assist the participants with any aid.

There was a gentleman who sat beside me who forgot to bring running socks, and his were obviously soaked from the bike ride. Because I was redundant in my preparation I brought along 2 pairs of socks in my transition bag and gave him one of my extra pairs. The blister that can result from wet socks, especially in a marathon, can ruin anyone's race. I was glad to help out a fellow rookie Ironman participant.

Also at T2 I had a zip-lock bag of race essentials that I brought along during my previous half-Ironman events. Antiseizure medication was a necessity; Advil, salt tabs, and glucose tabs were also among its contents. I would judiciously consume what I needed along the way, if there was any sign of cramping, fatigue or the slightest premonition of a seizure.

By the time I was out of T2, the race clock read 7 hours and 41 minutes, and that was the biggest shot of confidence for me the entire day. Knowing that the fastest athletes had not yet finished was exciting, too. I was nearly three miles into the run when I finally saw the two leaders alongside each other. Knowing that I was on the run portion a half hour before the fastest athletes would finish was exhilarating. At that point the possibility of finishing the Ironman under 12 hours seemed like a real possibility. Maybe . . . just maybe.

Aid stations for the run were approximately a mile apart from each other.

I contained my excitement as I embarked on the marathon course. My legs were heavy from the bike but not worn. My game plan was still intact. Never miss an opportunity to eat, enjoy the day, and have fun, and I was doing exactly that. The out-and-back running course through Penticton and to the south side of Skaha Lake and back wasn't as flat as I remembered it from when I visited in 2009. It was contoured with rolling hills.

I remained upbeat as much as possible whenever I passed other runners by saying, "Nice work" or "You're doing amazing," or "Keep it up." I would often say the same thing if runners passed me. I learned from previous races that encouragement to fellow athletes throughout the course of competition was important for my self morale.

Around mile 7 on the run, I passed a tandem team who had a leash wrapped around their waists. They had passed me on the bike leg around mile 60, and I never caught with them until this point. I observed that one of them had a prosthetic leg, and I became inspired.

I had a pair of tube socks in my special needs bag at the turnaround point of the marathon. The toes were cut off so I could use them as arm warmers. Since it rained during the bike leg, the possibility of showers loomed during the run. At times it sprinkled lightly but never rained to the extent it did climbing Yellow Lake. I was sure glad to have those throwaway socks. Everything else that I would need for the second half of the marathon was either already in my pocket or could be provided at the mile markers.

With all of Dave Fish's Ironman experience, I never thought that I would finish an Ironman race before him. He had an aggravated calf issue that bothered him all summer, and it became most evident during the run at Ironman Canada. I caught up to him at around mile 14 and walked along side him asking if there was anything he needed. I offered a couple of Advil that were in my special needs bag, which he accepted just in case. I pressed on.

As I got deeper into the marathon, I felt stronger and stronger. I was ultra conservative on the first half. By the time I was at mile 16, I started to pick up the pace, just as Dave recommended on that day of revelation around Donner Lake. Each aid station was an opportunity to re-energize, and for the first time on the course, one of the aid stations served warm chicken broth. I had been consuming pretzels, gels, oranges, banana slices, water, and Gatorade along the run course, but the chicken broth was the best. My body responded immediately to the sodium intake.

With six miles to go, the race wasn't getting any easier, but I was in high spirits. I didn't struggle during the marathon, and if I needed a break I would walk. Since the marathon course was an out-and-back, it was nice to see landmarks and streets that I ran along on the way out. When I got to downtown, I remembered approximately where the two leaders had passed me on my way out as they were running back in. I could not wait to get to that finish line.

Sure my legs were fatigued, and at times I could feel pulses of cramping along the final miles. But I was getting close, and I knew I would be finished in less than 30 minutes with 3 miles to go. Heck, I felt I could run an additional 10 more miles if the course was built for it. It was at that point I mentally finished the race and my body needed to catch up with my ego.

At the beginning of the run, there is an out-and-back section that runs about a half mile along Lakeshore Drive, east and west. To finish the course, athletes must retrace that same path, which is just shy of a mile. This was significant because the second half of the marathon is northbound. The mental shift back to east and west signaled that the end of the race was very near. I wasn't overwhelmed with emotion because I already visualized the outcome in my head, but it was a sense of relief knowing that I was less than a mile from becoming an Ironman.

My emotional highlights of the race occurred during the bike leg and when I saw the finish line before me at 11 hours, 57 minutes. It was surreal. I sprinted to the end with everything I had. *Danny Heinsohn, you are an Ironman!* is what I heard on the PA. Each finisher was greeted by two race supporters who wrapped each person in a space blanket. They were trained to make sure the athletes were feeling OK; if nutrition or medical support was needed, they would provide it. My mom and Michelle's family weren't too far away, as I found them within ten minutes along the guardrail and hugged my mom tightly. We later hit the massage tent, where I was worked on by two therapists for a half hour. By the time I was out, it was dark, and I regrouped with my mom and put on a pair of long running pants and the gray hoodie I bought at Walmart.

I knew it was only a matter of time before Michelle would cross the finish line, so I brought my camera to the home stretch and waited. I spotted her and took pictures as she crossed and yelled, "You're awesome, Michelle!" She finished around 10:30 p.m. We regrouped after she met with Brian and the rest of her family, and I gave her a hug. Not long after, my mom and I headed back to the Carmi Inn. I slept uninterrupted for nearly 12 hours. It was one of the best night's sleep I ever had. I couldn't have been happier.

MONDAY, AUGUST 30, 2010

My mom and I returned to the expo for my one-hour massage. It was amazing, but I still limped afterward. I was reminded of my experience at registration in 2009 for the 2010 Ironman Canada, as I observed the long line that went from the registration tent to several blocks out along the sidewalk. It was humbling. That evening my mom and I would enjoy a protein-and-pasta-packed dinner with Dave Fish, his girlfriend Nancy Thiele, Keith Juhola, and his wife, Shell.

I asked Dave and Keith if they remembered the tandem team whom I past on the run at about mile seven. Dave replied, "Yeah, one guy had a prosthetic leg and the other guy was blind".

TUESDAY, AUGUST 31, 2010

On the way back to Spokane, my mom and I picked up coffee at a gas station along with a couple copies of the Penticton Herald. One copy was for Michelle Morck, which I mailed to her after I returned home. The newspaper listed all of the finishers along with their times. I finished the Ironman competition with an official time of 11:57:24. I placed 897 out of over 3000 registered athletes and finished with the fastest time for the state of Nevada.

The coffee buzz during the drive left me wide-eyed and euphoric as we drove to Oliver to pick up some bottles of wine. Along the drive I had a vision similar to what I experienced when my family and I returned home from UCLA in 1999. My mission in life was drawn out and defined before me. I wanted to become a motivational speaker, raise money to help young cancer survivors get back on their feet, be an advocate for survivorship, and coordinate awesome experiences through sports marketing initiatives. This was my calling.

My Ironman dream had come true, I conquered brain cancer, started my own foundation, and exceeded my $10,000 fund-raising goal for My Hometown Heroes.

Mom and I returned to Reno later that evening, and I was back to work at Access Pass & Design the following day.

THE REST OF 2010 WAS A CELEBRATION

When I returned to the office at Access Pass & Design on Wednesday, there were posters of me all over the office. Bill superimposed my 5-year remission race photo onto a Wheaties box with my Ironman finish time at the bottom. Various fruits with my Ironman finish time of 11:57:24 were arranged on paper plates. The "11" was two bananas, "57" was done in blueberries, and "24" was spelled out in raspberries. I shared highlights of the day, as our team enjoyed fresh fruit, bagels, and cream cheese. It was pretty awesome, and I was grateful for the support from the Access family. Who would have predicted that meeting Seth in 2002 would lead to this?

Many of my friends were also anxious to congratulate me in person. My clients in the sports industry came up with their own versions of celebrating my accomplishment. The Seattle Seahawks had been a client of mine since 2009, and the director of media services loved working with Access's Bill Nutt. Two weeks following Ironman Canada, we flew to Seattle to visit our client for the first time, and we were granted field access for pregame warm-ups. They played the San Francisco 49ers, who went on to prevail.

THE YANKEES – 2010

The following week I was in New York for the Sports Marketing Symposium and client meetings. Michael Margolis of the New York Yankees was up to speed on my Ironman and philanthropic achievements, and he was able to fulfill and invitation request for three guests and me to a Yankees game. At the time the Yankees were in heated contention for the AL East title with the Tampa Bay Rays. That game would be a sellout.

Before leaving for New York, Michael mentioned in a phone call that there would be a special treat for Access Pass & Design during the game. During batting practice, Michael pulled me to the side and said, "In the middle of the third inning, we're going to welcome Access Pass & Design on the scoreboard."

Bonner Paddock was in town for the conference, so naturally I invited him. Navigate Marketing President A. J. Maestas was a National Sports Forum alumnus, and he was also in the city. I invited the two of them, along with the vice president of a global marketing agency based in New York. We enjoyed the prime on-field viewing experience in the close company of Derek Jeter, Reggie Jackson, A-Rod, Jorge Posada, CC Sabathia, and a candid Joe Girardi.

A lot of our clients refer to our company as Access Passes, which is also our website URL. I was able to meet Michael and a few of my other Yankees contacts on the field before the end of batting practice. My guests and I later enjoyed dinner at the New York Yankees steak house, where I excused myself and walked outside at the beginning of the third inning to take a snapshot of the New York Yankees greeting which read Yankees Welcome Access Passes.

Client appreciation doesn't get much better than that.

MORE POST-IRONMAN FUN

Three weeks following my visit to New York I found myself in Charlotte to attend my first NASCAR race at Charlotte Motor Speedway: the Bank of America 400. My client at GMR Marketing invited me to hang out on the track infield to network, meet with industry peers, and have a great time. I would watch the race with my clients on the Coors Light Party Deck.

Two days later the TEAMS conference began with a golf scramble followed by venue tours and an opening reception at Charlotte Motor Speedway, where Richard Petty Racing offered three-lap ride-alongs on the track for $99. I participated and chose the car of my biggest brand client, Miller Lite. We reached an exhilarating top speed of 160 miles per hour, and I gained a new appreciation for the sport.

Jesse Viner's wedding would be in January 2011, and his bachelor party took place in mid-December in Chicago. Attendees included Jesse, his childhood friends Brad and Max, and me. It began with a classic NHL rivalry at the United Center between the Chicago Blackhawks and Detroit Red Wings. I had just secured the Blackhawks account after they won the Stanley Cup earlier that year, and we got great seats. The Blackhawks would prevail that evening, 4 to 3.

2010 was an epic year.

A MOMENT TO REFLECT
Life Lessons from 10 Years of Survivorship

The second five years of remission were the most exciting times of my life. I turned 30 at the beginning of that period. The fruits of my labor through my professional, personal, and philanthropic life began to blossom. Through Access Pass & Design, I began working with the biggest teams and brands in the land including the New York Yankees, Minnesota Vikings, Lucas Oil Racing, Chicago Blackhawks, Visa, Red Bull, and Nike.

The Reno endurance community inspired me to coach over 40 people to ride their first century bike ride through *Team in Training*. During that time we raised over $125,000 for the Leukemia & Lymphoma Society. I ran my first marathon during that time and competed in several triathlons.

Everything came together between 2009 and 2010 but it was through the mentorship and inspiration of others that I was able to realize my true potential. My Hometown Heroes became the byproduct of all of this.

TEN LESSONS FROM TEN YEARS
- Great ideas are only great if they are put into action.
- For different results, change the way you think.
- True friendships endure the test of time.
- Be thankful for what you have.
- When it comes to business, story telling is the most valuable form of currency.
- You can't expect the unexpected.
- Take the time to reflect and be proud of what you've accomplished.
- Encourage others and give back.
- Leadership is action, not position.
- If you can influence, you can lead.

CHAPTER 25

SURVIVORSHIP IS A LIFESTYLE

USA Triathlon posted the All-American list in their 2010 rankings at the begin-ning of 2011. Based on their point system I ranked 1805 out of 3135 with a total of 71.91656 points in the 30-34 age group. The highest ranking was 102.3549 and the lowest was 32.86015. It felt good to be named an All-American.

2011 – INTO A NEW FRONTIER

All triathletes have their own reasons to compete in the 140.6-mile endur-ance event. For some it's a profession, for others it's a lifestyle, or a challenge to test themself. My reason was to celebrate life, ten years of survivorship, and to show appreciation to all who supported and inspired me throughout the years.

The journey brought me a renewed sense of self and revealed my calling in life. Throughout my training and creating My Hometown Heroes, I real-ized that I had become an agent of change. There was a mission and purpose behind everything I was motivated to do. I was passionate, persistent, and determined. But life after Ironman Canada wasn't happily ever after. I had my work cut out for me.

There is a term referred to as Post-Ironman Depression Syndrome (PIDS). When you dedicate 12 consecutive months of your life (several years for some) to train for an Ironman triathlon, sacrifices are made, and other life priorities slow down or are put on hold to make way for the Ironman dream. Training for the Ironman, working a full-time job, starting up a nonprofit, losing my father, and taking care of my mom in 2010 took me far beyond my comfort zone. Training for the Ironman was truly like working a second full-time job. When that routine ended, I certainly enjoyed the simplicity of returning to a much less regimented lifestyle.

Training for Ironman Canada became my coping mechanism to distract me from my father's passing in 2010. When that distraction dissolved and 2011 came around, dormant emotions reawakened and often engulfed me at unsuspecting times. I had to come to terms with my feelings and let the process run its course.

My new business development momentum at the beginning of 2010 evaporated as I dealt with the loss of my dad, and my primary focus shifted to Ironman training. My sales were down by nearly 25 percent in the first and second quarters of 2011. It wasn't because my clients went anywhere as much as it was they diverted their spending to different projects that wouldn't require the use of our services. When training for the Ironman, I was merely keeping afloat in my sales efforts and going through the motions instead of rowing out to new opportunities.

A couple of my friends with whom I trained for century bike rides and marathons began their own online marketing businesses in 2010. With all the attention I was getting from my Ironman accomplishment, they propositioned me with opportunities to work with them. I gave both businesses a shot, as I saw opportunities that those platforms could benefit My Hometown Heroes and my business at Access Pass & Design. But after a few months it became apparent that my attention to the new ventures was just too much for me to handle. I was doing everything half-ass, and in order for them to begin to grow, it required me to take more focus away from Access, which was where I needed to focus the most. After about three months I relinquished those opportunities to free up my time and channel my focus back to Access.

I turned to a couple of friends of similar age and career success, and I asked if they knew any therapists that could help me navigate through the tough times. My friend Dave White highly recommended someone he turned to as he began to take on more sophisticated responsibilities in his career. We were in the Denver airport at the time, waiting for our flight back to Reno after a Linkin Park concert at the Pepsi Center.

Dave's therapist was Dr. Diana Wright, and I called her office upon my return from Denver and scheduled an appointment. I came into the session with an open mind and gave her a general overview of my recent past with the Ironman achievement, the passing of my father, and my desire to finish writing my book.

She moved me to tears during that first visit. All of the memories about my dad were positive and joyful, and the more I talked about him, the more I realized how much I missed him and began to cry. Dr. Wright mentioned, "He really loved you."

I felt great comfort in those words, and it helped me realize I still needed to give myself time to heal. I would see Dr. Wright every few weeks. Some sessions were more productive than others, but they all served as stepping-stones to bring me closer to finding resolution. One day in the spring she said, "You keep mentioning your book. That's really important to you. I think what you need to do is take your book and move it to the top of your priority list."

She continued, "Set aside time during every week that's dedicated to you finishing your book. If you don't feel like writing, sit in front of your computer during those allocated times so you're in the right space, and when inspiration strikes you can take advantage." And so I did. I began allocating block-out time in the fall of 2011 and remained faithful. My goal was to have the book finished by the end of 2012 and published by 2013.

During this time of discovery I maintained my fitness base and began to train for the Eugene Marathon which would take place in May. My goal time was to finish under 3:30, which would have been a PR by over 10 minutes since the Las Vegas Marathon at the end of 2009. I PR'd Eugene by nearly 20 minutes with a time of 3h 23m 38s.

Business at Access began to take a turn for the better for me in the third and fourth quarters. In the fall of 2010 I pitched a proposal to the owners to begin an internship program to grow our business in the college football space. I concocted a highly effective marketing strategy in 2007 that has been yielding an average 400 percent return on investment annually. I realized this was a strategy that could be easily taught and managed by a college intern, especially one who had a passion for sports. We hired an enthusiastic gentleman named Kyle Fleming, who served five years in the army and had seen action in Afghanistan. He was in his second semester at Nevada. In late March we hit the ground running, and our campaign yielded a 500 percent return in new college football business.

I shared everything I could with Kyle about my experience in sports marketing and social media. I got him tuned up with the basics on Twitter and LinkedIn. Kyle is now a staple in our marketing department. In sharp contrast to the first two quarters, my year in sales ended up at a little over break-even, which meant growth in the third and fourth quarters was up by 50 percent.

My proudest achievement of 2011 was the opportunity to award the first scholarship of My Hometown Heroes. Recipient Kristen Katich and I stayed in touch since my Ironman finish when I made a promise to her: she would throw the first pitch at the Reno Aces baseball game on May 13. I also purchased tickets for her entire family to attend.

As fate would have it, Kristen's mom, Leslie, was the program director for the Northern Nevada Children's Cancer Foundation (NNCCF). She got involved not long after Kristen was diagnosed. I found great joy in this level of involvement, and I wanted to do more.

2012

Access Pass & Design grew by 24 percent in 2012, and I had a personal record-breaking year in sales at nearly 35 percent growth over 2011. In fact the entire company enjoyed 24% overall growth that year. I traveled over 40,000 miles for work within the continental United States, which was a record for me in a 12-month period. It wasn't by choice as much as it was for business development opportunities.

I spent a week on vacation in Alaska in July. It was my first real vacation in nearly three years, which was way too long to go without one, and I certainly didn't consider Ironman Canada to be a vacation. I made a personal vow to myself from that point forward to always take a vacation every year.

My Hometown Heroes received non-profit 501c3 status at the end of May, so that was something worth celebrating as much as it was a relief. The organization had awarded two recipients and contributed to families whose lives were affected by cancer.

I finished writing my book manuscript on 12/12/12, the same day I was sent to a Rapport leadership retreat by Access Pass & Design. And so, the editing process had begun.

RESOLVE

When I awakened after my second craniotomy in May 1999, I wasn't sure what my future would hold. I couldn't see straight, I slurred my words when I spoke, I barely knew who or where I was. I learned that a portion of my skull that was larger than a baseball card was no longer there, and a portion of my brain the size of a racquetball had been removed. But there was a buzz that lingered in my head to fill the void, and it never went away. As the years went on this buzz became my calling.

Thoughts were racing and colliding into each other during my days in the hospital and they persisted when I returned home. I couldn't sit still, nor could I get a good night's sleep. I thought I might go insane if I didn't act upon the calling but I found salvation and purpose through family and friends.

At the time I could not write by hand because the seizure after the first craniotomy short-circuited that motor function. Friends recommended that I begin keeping a journal, and I began typing my thoughts on the computer by one slow keystroke at a time with my index fingers. But it was a great way to keep the neurons in my head active. Slowly but surely my mind and body found a way to rewire and function together as one. That was hard to believe at first but staying active, I learned, is an essential ingredient to longevity.

When I finished writing my essay in October 1999 it became my gift to friends, family, and doctors. Nearly fourteen years later I have written a book, which will now be my gift to the world.

Everything happens for a reason. But what matters most is our friends and family. When times are tough, we lean on our loved ones and the community for comfort and support. Through them we find reason to carry on through the tough times. Through them we find inspiration.

If it weren't for Team in Training and the Leukemia & Lymphoma Society I would have never met Dan Brown, who guided me around Lake Tahoe on that hallowed day in 2001. If I didn't choose to become a spinning instructor I might not have ever met Seth Sheck from Access Pass & Design. If I didn't meet Lisa Furfine at the TEAMS conference in August of 2004 I may have never learned about the National Sports Forum. If I didn't attend Dan Migala's breakout session in 2007 I'm not so sure I would have found the success I did in the sports industry. If Bonner Paddock never climbed Mount Kilimanjaro to start his own foundation I may not have been as motivated to start my own foundation to celebrate ten years of survivorship. If it wasn't for the ongoing love, support, and inspiration of friends and family, I may not have been inspired to write this book.

At the beginning of the Fall 2013 semester, My Hometown Heroes awarded six young adult cancer survivors with scholarships of $1000 and $1500 each. By the time my 20th year of remission comes around my hope is to have raised enough money to award $1,000,000 in scholarship money to the young adult cancer survivor population.

To learn how you can help me reach that goal:
Check out www.myhometownheroes.org, follow on Twitter, and Like on Facebook.